COPING WITH PROSTATE CANCER RECURRENCE

MICHAEL J. DATTOLI, MD

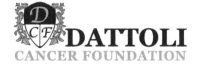

DATTOLI
CANCER FOUNDATION

SARASOTA, FLORIDA

Prostate Cancer Essentials for Survival Series: Coping with Prostate Cancer Recurrence

Copyright © 2022 by Michael J. Dattoli

ISBN-10: 1-7242781-6-9
ISBN-13: 978-1-7242-7816-6

Published by the Dattoli Cancer Foundation, Sarasota, FL
Imprint of record: CreateSpace, Charleston, SC
Book design and composition by Dan van Loon, Batavia, IL

MEDICAL DISCLAIMER

This book is intended as a supplement but not as a substitute for the medical advice of a physician. It is imperative that you consult a qualified healthcare professional with regard to all matters relating to your health and particular situation. Neither the publisher nor the authors bear responsibility for any consequences due to the reader's decision to use any particular treatment, medication, or other healthcare practices discussed in this book.

DEDICATION

This booklet is dedicated to all those whose lives have been touched by prostate cancer, and to the patients and their families whom we are privileged to serve and educate as cancer care providers.

ACKNOWLEDGMENTS

We are deeply grateful to a number of people who have contributed to this booklet in a number of ways. Our thanks to Greg Lawrence, for his editorial efforts and to Ginya Carnahan, Chris Wells, and Jone Fay at the Dattoli Cancer Center & Brachytherapy Research Institute for their ongoing assistance.

We deeply appreciate all of those wonderful patients and family members who have contacted the Dattoli Cancer Foundation for counseling and guidance and in turn have given us their support and encouragement. It is your spirit and commitment in confronting this disease that inspires us all.

CONTENTS

VIGILANCE
IS THE PATH
TO VICTORY

Virtually all patients who have been treated for prostate cancer live with the possibility that their cancer will reappear at some point in the future. There is some risk of relapse or recurrence over time regardless of the type of treatment or the stage of the cancer when the disease was first diagnosed. Of course, the best outcome with regard to relapse is not to have one, because your initial primary treatment is the best shot for a cure. A properly staged patient who takes advantage of the most advanced diagnostic modalities and chooses the most appropriate treatment for his case stands the best chance of avoiding relapse. Since there is no perfect treatment, there will always be some cases of recurrence, but the good news is that all treatments for prostate cancer, including salvage therapy for recurrence, have greatly improved in recent years.

While the likelihood of the disease reappearing diminishes with each passing year after initial treatment, as part of a prostate cancer battle plan, it is important for patients to be aware of their options down the line if a relapse should occur. With that knowledge, patients can be empowered to more effectively cope with any contingency. Some men may prefer to ignore the situation until a problem arises, but in the case of recurrence, they will face the task of doing their research and evaluating their treatment options under the emotional duress of the disease as it progresses. Playing ostrich is no way to fight prostate cancer.

Patients are therefore advised to explore their options for further treatment in advance and think through a tentative plan of action to pursue if the need should ever arise. Knowing their options and being prepared for any eventuality can enable patients to have peace of mind about their health. There is no need to be taken unaware or shocked as most patients are when first diagnosed. Fortunately, for most patients who have to face the disease again, there are still courses of treatment available regardless of which treatment they underwent in the past. Depending on a man's age and the stage of his disease, recurrence of prostate cancer for some patients may not be life-threatening and may not require further treatment. Keep in mind that it is never patients who fail, but rather treatments that sometimes fail to completely eradicate the disease. Treatment failure means that a particular form of therapy has not been successful in fully eliminating the cancer or in controlling the progression of the disease.

If you are facing recurrence, above all else, don't beat yourself up for the treatment choice you made originally. In the language of urology, the physician will say "you failed," when in fact it was the treatment that failed you. You must not fault yourself for the decision you made. That was then; this is now.

When evaluating treatment failure, doctors determine whether the failure is "local," "regional" or "distant." A local failure indicates the cancer has reappeared in the area of the prostate (or in the prostate bed, if the gland was removed by surgery). A regional failure indicates the spread of disease is still confined to the prostate and pelvic region. Distant failure indicates there are metastases at sites in the body distant from the prostate, such as lymph nodes or bones. In some cases, there may only be evidence of biochemical recurrence (a rising PSA). Determining whether treatment failure is local or distant is crucial in deciding what options each patient has for future therapy, and whether or not additional therapy is appropriate. A distant failure may not be a recurrence per se, but rather an indication of persistent disease that was not detected during the initial workup and staging. In such cases, the cancer was probably there before the primary treatment but not detected by the various diagnostic scans and lab tests.

It is important to understand at this point that treating a recurrence is more challenging than initially treating most prostate cancers, whether the relapse is local, regional or distant. There will be a new set of critical circumstances to consider. Primary among these is the condition of the prostate bed or the prostate gland (if first treatment was anything other than surgery). Surgery (either open radical or robotic) leaves a void in the pelvic area that rapidly becomes occupied by the bladder and/or rectum, making radiation tricky so as not to permanently damage these organs in the process of killing the remaining cancer cells. In addition, the surgical process will have left the area badly devascularized (decreased blood flow), therefore–the "target zone" will be lacking in appropriate oxygenation to activate the highest killing response for radiation. Higher doses, only achieved by **DART**, Dynamic Adaptive Radiotherapy, often accompanied by hormonal therapy, are necessary as salvage therapy with these post-surgical cases, which are indeed becoming epidemic.

This booklet will discuss the available options for local, regional, and distant failure after each type of mainstream primary therapy. Before deciding on any second course of treatment, you should fully investigate the likelihood of eradicating the cancer and the risk of side effects that may alter your quality of life. These are the most important considerations in deciding on salvage therapy. Given your age and overall health, you will want to find a balance between effectiveness and side effects—a balance with which you are comfortable, that you can live with both before and after treatment. Knowing what to expect each step of the way is one of the keys to fighting this disease.

The shared goal of the Dattoli Cancer Team with this booklet is to help you make *informed decisions* about your treatment. Don't delegate those decisions to someone else. After all, it's your body and your health that are at stake. As you gather information, always consider the source and use your own judgment about your personal needs. *You will ultimately know best what is right for you.* If this is your second time around with prostate cancer, don't be afraid to voice your concerns to your doctor and don't hesitate to ask questions—you have every right to know the answers and to expect a standard of care with which you are satisfied.

RECENT PROGRESS WITH DIAGNOSING AND TREATING RECURRENT PROSTATE CANCER

More than fifteen years ago, we published the first edition of this booklet (*Prostate Cancer Recurrence: Need You Be Concerned?*) and later an article in the Spring 2012 issue of *Journey*, (a a donor-supported publication from the Dattoli Cancer Foundation) entitled "New Options in Metastatic Prostate Cancer Treatment." At that time, Provenge® (sipuleucel-T), a form of immunotherapy, had recently been approved by the FDA and was finding its way to patients with advanced and recurrent prostate cancer who had exhausted both hormone therapy and chemotherapy. While the reported overall survival improvement with the drug was only four months, this positive development gave new hope to many patients who had few options and were facing grim prospects at that time.

We have come a long way since then. Research developing Provenge® soon led to a number of similar prostate cancer immunotherapeutic drugs that have also won FDA approval. As we will discuss later in this booklet, other novel therapeutic agents are now being regularly prescribed for hormone-refractory prostate cancer (see below, "What Options Are Available Once Hormonal Therapy Stops Working?").

Looking back over these seven years, in addition to new drugs, we have seen some interesting trends in both diagnosis and treatment of prostate cancer. We believe one of these is the unfortunate byproduct of a recommendation first made by the U.S. Preventive Services Task Force (USPSTF) in 2012 (and updated in 2018) that has discouraged men from getting routine PSA blood tests, and is predictably resulting in more men presenting with advanced cancer to lymph nodes and bone beyond the prostate gland than previously seen (Lee, DJ, Recent changes in prostate cancer screening practices and prostate cancer epidemiology, J Urol. 2017 May 25).[1] Yet another alarming trend is the dramatic increase in numbers of men coming to us very shortly after having robotic surgery (robotic radical prostatectomy), reporting that their PSA never fell following surgery or if it did fall, it soon began to climb again and did so rapidly in many cases. These are men who believed that robotic surgery would resolve their prostate cancer threat with fewer side effects than conventional prostatectomy ("open retropubic").

These cases are not strictly recurrence per se, but are more correctly termed prostate cancer persistence. Their initial, original treatment did not remove all of their prostate cancer, and a secondary treatment (radiation or hormones or both) is required. If we see these men early enough following surgery (the lower the PSA, the better) we have had good success in defeating their cancers, once and for all, utilizing salvage Dynamic Adaptive Radiation Therapy (DART) to maximally avoid unwanted toxicities to neighboring critical organs and structures. Perhaps if we had seen them first, our combination external radiation therapy coupled with brachytherapy, most likely would have totally eliminated their disease in the first place, and the patient could have been spared the side effects of surgery. Nonetheless, surgery remains an option in select patients following advanced diagnostic staging.

One encouraging observation with regard to these patients with persistent disease is that the word is finally getting through to urologists and oncologists that as soon as the PSA starts to rise, the patient should be evaluated for further treatment. In the recent past, these men (the patients and their physicians) often waited until the PSA was up around 2.0 or higher before any action was taken. Today we know that if the PSA inches up to even 0.2, or two consecutive rises after surgery (even if less than 0.2), one should start considering further treatment (radiation +/- hormones). Recognize that prostate cancer recurrence following surgery may be comprised of high grade, mutated, undifferentiated cancers which bear little resemblance to normal prostate cancer cells. In view of this, these cancers often flourish and yet produce minimal amounts of PSA.

So what is in store for the man whose rising PSA following surgery signals the recurrence or persistence of his prostate cancer? The first step is to verify the presence of disease, and whether it is local (in the "prostate bed"–tissue left behind) or beyond the prostate or both. Newer, more sophisticated diagnostic technologies can determine the location (-s) of recurrent/persistent malignancy, whether the cancer is still confined to the prostate bed or has spread to the lymph nodes or bones.

After a thorough review of the recurrent patient's history and current lab and imaging reports, ruling out local or regional extension of the disease (meaning the immediate area outside the prostate gland), we may recommend an advanced lymph node screening exam as well as screening for metastatic disease spread to bone and visceral organs. Prior to 2009, these men were sent to the Netherlands for a Combidex scan, which utilizes nanoparticles as a contrast agent for Magnetic Resonance Imaging (MRI) to detect distant prostate cancer spread.

For almost ten years, we have been sending men with suspected distant metastatic disease for another nanoparticle test called Ferumoxytol (Feraheme) which has high predictive accuracy to detect lymph node disease. This test is most commonly coupled with an 18F PET/CT scan, a very exacting test for detecting disease spread to bone. These nanoparticle tests are known as USPIO scans (ultra-small super paramagnetic iron oxide) or Feraheme, referring to the reagent used in imaging. For this test, the patient is injected with the reagent one day, and the scan is performed the next day (Dattoli MJ, et al, Efficacy of Ferumoxytol (Feraheme) as a Lymphatic Contrast Agent in Prostate Cancer, ASCO 2018 Genitourinary Cancer Symposium, February 8-10, 2018).

The reagent used will "light up" the lymph chain and clearly indicates which nodes are harboring active prostate cancer cells. With this information, we can design precision DART treatments to address those specific lymph nodes and treat them to a high dose level. Since the test is based on advanced CT and MRI imaging, visceral metastasis to liver and lung can also be detected.

Other advanced imaging tests include PET/CT C-11 Choline and PET/CT Carbon Acetate C-11 scans. Aside from nanoparticle imaging, other functional and molecular imaging is being carried out. For example, Gallium-68 PSMA (Ga-68) is being investigated and has great promise. It attaches to PSMA which is on the surface of metastatic prostate cancer cells and can therefore detect bone, lymph node and visceral metastases with high predictive accuracy, even with low PSA's. Because Ga-68 is much more stable than C-11 Choline (which is short lived and has to be made one dose at a time at select imaging centers), the Ga-68 PSMA test could be used at medical centers around the nation (Hofman MS, Gallium-68 Prostate-Specific Membrane Antigen PET Imaging, PET Clin, 2017 Apr;12(2):219-234).

Meanwhile, 3D Color-Flow Power Doppler Ultrasonography (used at our center and a few select centers worldwide) can pick up intra-prostatic cancer recurrence after radiotherapy. The Dattoli Team has reseeded more than 1,000 patients with intact prostates with great success and limited morbidity. This is referred to as a salvage prostate cancer treatment (either partial prostate or entire prostate). Other potential salvage options include, but are not limited to, cryosurgery (freezing), HIFU (heating), biothermy (freezing and heating), and focal MRI-guided interstitial ablation. Each has its own potential benefit and side effect profile.

Any of the above therapies can treat the entire prostate gland or a portion of the gland (i.e. partial treatment). Partial treatment should never be recommended as initial treatment and should only be considered as salvage therapy. Similar to breast cancer, prostate cancer is also a "field effect" disease. That is, what has happened at one or several locations in the prostate will occur elsewhere in the gland since all cells have been subject to the same environmental cues and genetic predilections. This will lead to multiple future focal treatments and greatly increased morbidity.

Most patients who recur in the prostate gland will be identified to have spread to other sites following careful re-staging. Even if the re-staging proves negative, we most often combine salvage re-seeding along with DART to the relevant nodal chains to cover the possibility that lymph nodes harbor microscopic cancer. To date, even the most sophisticated, advanced diagnostic tests cannot identify and locate microscopic disease.

We have been collecting data on these cases, namely men having lymph node and boney disease spread, and we have published articles in medical journals to report our success in utilizing Feraheme to detect lymph node spread. We are working with the University of Washington in Seattle and the results look extremely favorable. We are also using yet another advanced imaging test, 18F–Fluciclovine, more commonly known as an Axumin-Enhanced PET Scan, with impressive early results picking up residual recurrent disease within the prostate/prostate bed, lymph nodes, bones and visceral metastasis.

With regard to recurrence (and persistence), the message here again is that all men who have had a prostate cancer diagnosis and have been treated with any method should be very vigilant in watching their PSA. The moment the PSA starts to rise, attention should be given to the rise and finding out why it is rising. While drugs like Proscar and Avodart.are known to reduce the PSA, following prostate cancer diagnosis, many men take vitamin supplements and change their diets and lifestyles. This can be beneficial, with the objective to slow the rate of PSA rise, velocity, and doubling time, while improving the general health of patients.

There is, however, a scenario, especially with patients being followed under Active Surveillance whereby the PSA declines (without Avodart. or Proscar.) which may lull patients into a false sense of security. In patients following surgery, this is the often case since some cancers may mutate, become more aggressive, no longer resemble the parent prostate cell and are no longer even making PSA. This is a serious cause for concern. This phenomenon is often missed by urologists and oncologists.

Finally, it should be noted that in the same way that early diagnosis increases the likelihood of successful cure, the best time to treat a recurrence is as soon as it becomes evident.

What Is The "PSA Bounce"?

PSA bounce or PSA flare is a phenomenon experienced by about 30-40% of patients who have undergone prostate brachytherapy (seed implants) and 10-20% of patients receiving temporary High Dose Rate prostate brachytherapy (Makarewicz R, et al Jour Cont Brachy. 2009: 1(2) 92-96). While the most thoroughly analyzed patients are those having permanent seed implants, it has also been reported to occur in patients having undergone prostate irradiation alone to high dose level and we are even seeing this phenomenon occur in patients undergoing nodal radiation. It is a *temporary rise* in PSA usually occurring about 18 to 24 months following implant, possibly caused by radiation induced prostatitis (inflammation of the prostate which may be clinical and associated with prostate symptoms, or subclinical—that is, asymptomatic) triggering a release of PSA.

Interestingly, in approximately one third of these cases, there is no prostate inflammation. This is not either recurrence or persistence of prostate cancer, but a false alarm. The bounce seems to occur more often in younger men (55 years or younger), and in men of all ages having larger prostate glands. The PSA bounce may subside with a course of antibiotics or alpha-blockers or anti-inflammatory medications, or it may diminish naturally over time (Bernstein MB, et al, Prostate-specific antigen bounce predicts for a favorable prognosis following brachytherapy: a meta-analysis, J Contemp Brachytherapy: 2013 Dec; 5(4):210-4).

How is Recurrence Detected?

The methods used by doctors to monitor patients after primary treatment for prostate cancer include the ultrasensitive PSA blood assay, digital rectal exam, and additional follow-up testing, which may include a biopsy.

PSA Blood Assay

Since the late 1980s, the PSA blood assay has been widely used to monitor the progress of patients after treatment. The test determines the amount of prostate specific antigen circulating in the blood (measured in nanograms per milliliter, or ng/ml). At our institution, following radioactive seed implantation (brachytherapy) and/or Dynamic Adaptive Radiotherapy (DART, utilizing all the modalities associated with the most advanced Intensity Modulated Radiation Therapy, or 4-Dimensional Image-Guided IMRT), only patients who achieve and maintain a PSA nadir of 0.2 or less are considered disease-free. After seed implants and external radiation, the prostate is left in place and any remaining normal prostate cells will secrete PSA, so there will be a certain baseline PSA level.

We have patients with PSA levels as high as 3.0 that over time have never shown any PSA velocity (rate of increase of PSA). Their PSA readings have been fairly stable and not rising for a decade or more; however, when using strict 0.2 PSA nadir criteria, they are technically not considered cured or disease free, even though most of these patients will probably never have symptoms or die from prostate cancer. Therefore, most of them will not require further treatment.

Since the prostate gland is entirely removed by a radical prostatectomy, very little or no PSA should be found in the bloodstream if the surgery is successful. A PSA nadir value of 0.2 is often employed by surgeons. Any PSA reading higher than that would be indicative of treatment failure, also known as biochemical failure. With patients who had a Gleason score of 8 to 10 going into surgery, any rise should be taken quite seriously. This is the case since high grade tumors secrete little PSA and by the time the PSA reaches 0.2, the cancer burden may be quite high. These patients and their doctors should be especially cautious of any incremental rise of PSA even below the 0.2 nadir. Recent studies have suggested that a more cautious 0.1 nadir should be utilized for determining the success or failure of radical surgery, especially for higher risk patients (Hsu CC, et al, BJU Int. 2015 Nov;116(5):713-20.

We have known and advocated for more than two decades, that surgery is not a reasonable solution to prostate cancer because of the propensity of the disease to appear close to the gland margins and to grow aggressive microscopic fingers outside of the gland which cannot be removed with the surgical scalpel or by any robotic surgical technique.

Patients should be aware that their doctors may employ somewhat different PSA nadir criteria for evaluating the success of treatment. Be sure to question your physician carefully in this regard. If your PSA starts to rise, your doctor will probably want to check you more frequently, perhaps every 3 to 6 months to see if the trend continues. If the PSA value over time indicates biochemical failure, other tests will be used to determine whether or not the cancer is locally confined, regional or distant (metastatic disease). For the sake of consistency, the same PSA assay and lab should be used.

Reading and evaluating the PSA involves a sophisticated series of judgments, which are in turn evaluated in light of other tests. In younger patients with a rising

PSA, the likelihood is that some form of secondary treatment, or salvage therapy, will be indicated. With older patients, a slow PSA velocity or doubling time can sometimes mean that no further therapy will be necessary.

Patients are advised to check with their local laboratory to find out what brand of test is being used. You will want to be sure that the particular test at your lab has been FDA-approved for both diagnosis and monitoring of prostate cancer (as some tests are approved only for monitoring).

Additional Follow-up Testing

The digital rectal exam is also used for monitoring patients after primary treatment. This test is not the most reliable, but some recurrences can be detected with a DRE. The doctor will feel through the rectal wall for nodules or hardness or an enlargement of the prostate gland (if it hasn't been removed by surgery).

Other monitoring and follow-up testing can include a prostate biopsy, a bone scan, helical CT scan, ultrasound (preferably Color-Flow Power Doppler Ultrasound as well as conventional gray scale ultrasound), MRI (Magnetic Resonance Imaging, preferably Dynamic Contrast Enhanced MRI—or DCE-MRI—which is superior to any other MRI out there including the spectroscopic MRI), and other sophisticated fusion studies that combine techniques. As discussed previously, the use of encapsulated iron oxide nanoparticles or ultrasmall superparamagnetic iron oxide (USPIO) as MRI contrast agents is proving to be quite effective in identifying prostate cancer metastasis in the lymph nodes.

At our institution, we employ two Hitachi 3D Color-Flow Power Doppler Transrectal Ultrasound devices (3D-CFPD TRUS). What makes our Color doppler ultrasounds so special is the 3D power capability. We have documented a 97% predictive accuracy to diagnose prostate cancer (Dattoli et al, Prostate Biopsies using both gray scale and 3D Color-Flow Power Doppler Ultrasound (3D-CFPDU), ASCO-GU Symposium, February 2015). To improve on this capability, we are now fusing Multiparametric MRI images (utilizing a 3 Tesla magnet) and 3D-CFPDU. The yield has been 100% diagnostic accuracy.

When extensive lymph node involvement is detected, we use an arsenal of advanced techniques that define Dynamic Adaptive Radiotherapy, which allows us to follow the movement of organs and adjust for that natural motion. This allows us to zero in on the target while avoiding surrounding healthy tissue. This degree of accuracy is especially important when treating the pelvic lymph nodes. Here's where you really need to move away from conventional radiation, not 3D Conformal, not IMRT. DART is superior, and will be discussed in greater detail below.

Bone scans and CT scans often miss areas where the cancer is more occult. As noted, we also utilize 18F Flouride PET/CT fusion for detecting bone metastases. An Israeli study (Einat E et al., J Nucl Med 2006; 47:287-297) showed a 98% predictive accuracy for bones. It is also fairly accurate for lymph nodes. In addition, 11C-Choline PET/CT is currently being used at the Mayo Clinic. We also utilize the CTC (Circulating Tumor Cell) blood test, which provides information about the burden of cancer cells in the bloodstream.

Multiparametric and Dynamic Contrast Enhanced MRI calculates both increased vessel permeability and increased cellular density (also called extra-cellular volume), which are key physiological indicators of PCa. 75% accuracy has been reported with DCE-MRI (Bloch, et al, Radiotherapy Oncology, 2003, 66(2): 173-179). This is a very accurate test compared to pathological specimens taken during prostatectomy.

As illustrated on the back cover of this booklet, Color-Flow Power Doppler Ultrasound reveals suspicious red areas due to vascularity (blood flow). Normal tissues pulse with blood flow; cancers don't; they're stagnant, not in sync with the normal circu-lating blood flow. 3D Color-Flow Power Doppler Ultrasound is somewhat similar to Contrast Enhanced MRI. The two tests complement each other, as noted above.

At our institution, 3D Color-Flow Power Doppler Ultrasound is used to guide the biopsy needles in order to improve the likelihood of obtaining samples from potential tumor sites. As with the original diagnostic work-up that each patient has undergone, the purpose of all these follow-up tests is to determine the aggressiveness of the cancer and whether or not it has spread beyond the prostate region. If the cancer is locally confined, the patient is likely to be a candidate for some form of salvage therapy.

If the cancer has metastasized extensively (distant failure), some form of palliative treatment such as hormonal therapy is likely to be recommended (see "When Should Hormonal Therapy Be Initiated?"). When the cancer becomes hormone resistant, other agents and clinical trials may be recommended (see "What Options are Available Once Hormonal Therapy Stops Working?). Systemic disease is considered incurable, but that does not mean we don't treat it aggressively to try to control the disease and preserve quality of life as long as possible.

Patients with a limited number of metastases (lymph nodes and/or bone) have what is known as oligo-metastatic disease, and these patients may benefit from Dynamic Adaptive Radiotherapy (DART) in order to take these areas of disease out of the equation. Our ability to visualize these areas so we can aim at them has greatly improved in recent years. We believe we are giving these patients an additional lease on life and allowing them to preserve their quality of life as long as possible.

The Dattoli Team recently presented a a paper on USPIO imaging and treating oligo-metastatic disease in collaboration with the University California San Francisco (Dattoli MJ, et al, Radiotherapy guided by ultra small superparamagnetic iron oxide (USPIO)-contrast MRI staging for patients with advanced or recurrent prostate cancer. ACRO Radiation Oncology Summit, February 27-29, 2020). For more information on this subject, readers are referred to the Prostate Cancer Essentials booklet, Lymph Node Positive Prostate Cancer: Advanced Diagnostics and Treatment.

What Are The Risks Of Recurrence With Each Type Of Primary Treatment?

The likelihood of recurrence varies with the type of primary treatment and the number of years following treatment that a patient remains disease-free (as indicated by PSA and other monitoring tests). We will present in this section what we know about the probable outcomes for radiation therapy and radical surgery as the most utilized mainstream treatments.

There are two ways of looking at the contemporary prostate cancer literature and evaluating the risk of treatment failure (see Boxes 1 and 2). The first method stratifies patients according to low risk, intermediate risk and high risk groups. Low risk patients are generally defined as those who are less than or equal to Stage T2a, Gleason score less than or equal to 6, and PSA less than 10.0. Medium risk includes patients with Stage T2b or greater, Gleason Score equal to 7, and PSA of 10-20. High risk includes those patients with Stage T2c or greater, Gleason Score 8 to 10, and PSA greater than 20.

Another way of looking at risk stratification breaks down into favorable, intermediate and unfavorable groups. Stratification involves prognostication, meaning how well you will do with a particular treatment. Favorable risk features are Stage T2b or less, Gleason Score less than or equal to 6, and PSA less than 10. Intermediate would involve having two of the risk factors (Stage greater than T2b, Gleason Score greater than 6, and PSA equal to or greater than 10). Unfavorable would have all three risk factors.

Pre-treatment Risk Categories	% 5-year Failure Rate
Low Risk: Stage ≤ T$_{2a}$, Gleason 2-6, PSA<10	25%
Medium Risk: Stage T$_{2b}$, Gleason 7, PSA 10-20	>25 - 50%
High Risk: Stage T$_{2c}$, Gleason 8-10, PSA 2 20	>50%

Box 1: Likelihood of recurrence based on low, intermediate, and high risk for surgical patients, based on current NCCN (National Comprehensive Cancer Network) staging guidelines.

The Prostatic Acid Phosphatase (PAP) test is another indicator of risk, and we have done quite a bit of reporting on this test. PAP actually predated the PSA assay. Before the advent of PSA testing, doctors relied on the PAP test as an indicator of prostate cancer progression and prognosticator of whether or not patients would fail. In the pre-PSA era, patients would be told that they were not surgical candidates or curative treatment candidates if their PAPs were elevated. With the enthusiasm that came with the PSA test in the early 1990s, PAP wasn't as widely used. But we continued to use the PAP test in our research and came to find that it was in fact still important and perhaps more important than the PSA. Our findings are consistent with studies done at Johns Hopkins, Walter Reed Hospital, and by a large RTOG (Radiation Therapy Oncology Group) study.

OTHER RISK GROUP PROGNOSTICATION

Favorable: Stage $\leq T_{2a}$, Gleason 2-6, PSA < 10
Intermediate: 2 of the above indicators
Unfavorable: All 3 of the above indicators
Other: Elevated PAP (Prostatic Acid Phosphatase)

Box 2: Favorable, intermediate, and unfavorable risk stratification.

If you visit one of the nomogram websites, you can plug your own numbers into the prostate cancer arena to see where you stand in terms of risk. A nomogram is a graphic representation that can be used to analyze prostate cancer data. There are many nomograms including one for surgical patients created by Dr. Alan Partin at Johns Hopkins. He followed patients stratified by stage, PSA, and Gleason score who subsequently went on to have surgery, reporting how they fared, and thereby determining the risk of having extracapsular disease extension, meaning cancer that has extended beyond the prostate gland. When considering your own case, keep in mind that the outcomes are presented in terms of probabilities. The predictive power of nomograms is not absolute for any individual case, and in some cases, they may give flawed results.

As indicated in Box 3, a recent multicenter study citing research by Memorial Sloan Kettering Cancer Center estimates that 25,000 patients annually experience treatment failure (biochemical recurrence) after radical surgery, with 50% to 95% of high risk patients developing recurrence after surgery (Spratt DE, et al, Am Soc Clin Oncol Educ Book, 2018 May 23;(38):355-362).

We also know, as indicated in Box 4, that 13,500 patients annually will develop biochemical recurrence following primary radiation therapy, with 50% of those being in the initial high risk group (Mettlin, US Cancer, Vol. 86, 1999 and Stephenson, World J Urol, Vol. 15, 1997). This shouldn't be interpreted at face value to mean that radiation is doing better, because these are absolute numbers and there were more cases of surgery being followed than a 2013 study by Johns Hopkins researchers reported that 20–40% of patients undergoing radical prostatectomy and 30–50% of patients undergoing radiation therapy will experience biochemical recurrence within 10 years (Paller CJ, et al, Clin Adv Hematol Oncol. 2013 Jan; 11(1): 14–23). Results have improved with radiotherapy utilizing more advanced technology and combination techniques (Dattoli MJ, et al, "Long-term outcomes for patients with prostate cancer having intermediate and high-risk disease, treated with combination external beam irradiation and brachytherapy" Journal of Oncology, July 2010).

It should also be noted that there are more than 3 million men living today who have been treated for prostate cancer, and that number continues to grow. Long-term statistics resulting from other forms of treatment (such as Proton Beam Radiation Therapy (PBRT), HIFU, cryotherapy, Cyberknife®, Calypso, etc.) are not readily available, but will contribute to an even larger number of cases that recur.

Recurrence Following Prostatectomy

25,000 men per year will develop a biochemical recurrence) after Radical Prostatectomy.

Memorial Sloan Kettering Cancer Center, 2018

Box 3

Recurrence Following Primary Radiation

"13,500 patients will develop recurrence annually following primary irradiation (10% low-risk, 50% high-risk)."

Mettlin, US Cancer, Vol 86, 1999
Stephenson, World J Urol, Vol 15, 1997

Box 4

Patients should be aware that 25% to 50% of surgical patients who were thought to have disease contained within the prostate were later found to have cancer beyond the scope of the prostate. In the case of recurrence after radical prostatectomy, the patient may ask why is my PSA rising? It's all about location. Most prostate cancers begin in the peripheral zone, at the end of the gland. The prostate gland has no capsule per se to act a barrier against the dispersion of cancer cells outside the gland. We rarely find tumors in the central zone of the prostate.

Modern prostatectomy is a flawed cancer operation because it is not possible to obtain sufficient surgical margins, due to the proximity of 1) the prostate to the bladder, superiorly, 2) the rectum posteriorly, 3) the urogenital diaphragm inferiorly, and 4) the neurovascular bundles posterolaterally.

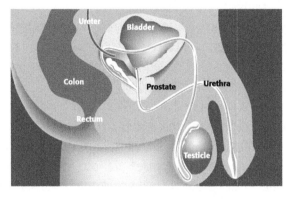

The challenge with treating prostate cancer surgically is the location of the gland within the context of surrounding organs.

We're seeing more and more prostate remnants left behind after surgery, especially laparoscopic and robotic techniques, and even residual seminal vesicles which should be gone after prostatectomy. Somehow the surgeon missed those crucial areas.

According to Fox Business News, despite the lack of both long-term data and compelling results, 92,000 Da Vinci robotic radical prostatectomies were performed in 2016 and that number is increasing. About 90% of all prostatectomies are now robotic even though the outcomes are at best only comparable to open surgery. Many patients are apparently being misled and victimized by the hype surrounding unproven surgical robotics.

In January 2017, a study favorably comparing robot-assisted to open surgery was published by researchers at Weill Cornell Medical College-New York Presbyterian Hospital. They offered their assessment of the field: "Robot-assisted surgery has been rapidly adopted in the U.S. for prostate cancer. Its adoption has been driven by market forces and patient preference, and debate continues regarding whether or not it offers improved outcomes to justify the higher cost relative to open surgery" (Hu JC, et al, J Urol. 2017 Jan; 197(1): 115-121).

While that study suggests a rough equivalence between the competing surgical techniques, we would argue from our point of view that market forces driven by advertising hype from medical centers and physicians without evidence-based data have contributed to misguiding many patients with regard to the as yet unproven advantages of robotic surgery.

A large study published in 2016 by the Mayo Clinic compared open, laparoscopic and robot-assisted radical prostatectomy with a 10-year patient follow-up. These

Can the Da Vinci Robotic Technique do better than the Open Retropubic?

Journal of Clinical Oncology, Vol 26, No 14, 2008 pp 2278-84 (Harvard Analysis)

"At 6 months, bio-chemical failure increased from 9.1% (open) to 27.8% (DaVinci robotic), with 40% increase in anastomatic strictures (DaVinci robotics)"

European Urology, Vol 54, No 4, 2008, pp 785-793 (Duke University)

"Patients who underwent robotic surgery had significantly higher levels of dissatisfaction and regret than patients undergoing retropubic radical prostatectomy."

European Urology, Vol 57, No 3, 2010, pp 363-550

"Patients undergoing MIRPs (minimally invasive radical prostatectomy) experienced 25% increased rates of incontinence and erectile dysfunction. "

Hu JC, et al, JAMA. 2009 Oct 14;302(14):1557-64.

"Is this just another way of cutting out the prostate? Approximately half of our patients at this point are those who have failed the robotic technique."

Michael J. Dattoli, M.D..

researchers reported that regardless of which surgical technique was utilized, serious urinary side effects and erectile dysfunction affected about 6.4% and 37.3% of patients respectively (Jackson MA, et al, Urology, May 2016, Volume 91, Pages 111–118).

Successful salvage radiation therapy depends on many factors. Primary among these is the location of the recurrence, whether the relapse is local (prostate bed, seminal vesicles, etc.) or distant (spine, lung, etc.).

As noted, more and more men are experiencing failure with robotic Da Vinci surgical removal. Because the gland itself is often mangled by the attempt to remove it using robotic techniques, these men are not usually eligible for seed implant. However, full course DART with 4D IG-IMRT is being offered to these men with confidence of efficacy, depending on the amount and location of positive cells, and the rapidity of diagnosis of recurrence.

We think it's significant that two studies have shown that without some form of salvage therapy 66% to 75% of patients with local recurrence will develop metastases within 10 years (see Box 5), and that is with or without hormonal therapy, also known as Androgen Deprivation Therapy, or ADT (Kella, et al, Amer J Urol Rev, 2004; Pound, et al, JAMA, 281, 1999). Extended survival is an important consideration

To recap, the problems with recurrence after radical prostatectomy are:

1. The target (the prostate and tumor) is no longer in place and this void becomes occupied by critical structures, particularly the bladder and rectum.

2. Because of this situation, only lower (suboptimal) doses can be achieved with conventional external radiation.

3. After surgery, the surgical bed is denuded of vessels (devascularized) and radiation works best in a vascularlized, oxygenated region. In theory, even higher doses are necessary than when the prostate is intact.

Solution
Only the sophistication of DART can achieve the required higher dose levels. Hormonal therapy is often used to "sensitize" the radiation to more effectively eradicate cancer.

because when we consider the projected expectancy of life, we are living longer than ever before. When a doctor is seeing a prostate cancer patient, he may use a 5 or 10 year rule of thumb for survival, assuming that if a patient has 5 or 10 years life expectancy, he shouldn't be treated because he is most likely to die from some other cause than his prostate cancer. But according to the latest statistics (Box 6), an 80-year-old man now has a life expectancy of almost 10 years. That's the average. If you happen to be a healthy 80-year-old, you're very likely to live more than 10 years. A healthy 90-year-old man is likely to live another 5 years. Given the overall trend, it is likely that increasing numbers of patients who experience treatment failure will be candidates for salvage therapy.

The numbers that we often see reported as deaths caused by prostate cancer are actually lower than the numbers in reality because many patients in their 70's and 80's are often discouraged from having curative treatments; rather they are given hormonal therapy. Over time, the hormonal therapy often makes patients fat, makes their bones weak, makes them anemic and may also cause cardiac problems (metabolic syndrome). A certain percentage of those patients will die from heart attacks or they may die from falling and developing stress fractures in their hips along with collateral bleeding. The reported cause of death may be heart attack or one of these other causes, when in fact the cause of death was really the culmination of long-term hormonal therapy for prostate cancer.

Salvage Radiation for Local Recurrence following Prostatectomy

Without salvage therapy 66-75% of men with local recurrence will develop bone metastasis within 10 years.

Pound, JAMA, Vol 281, 1999

Box 5

Projected Male Expectancy of Life: United States, 2018

AGE	AVG. LIFE EXPECTANCY
60	21.8 years
65	18.1
70	14.6
75	11.3
80	8.4
85	6.0
90	4.5

National Vital Statistics Reports, Vol. 69, No. 12, November 17, 2020

Box 6

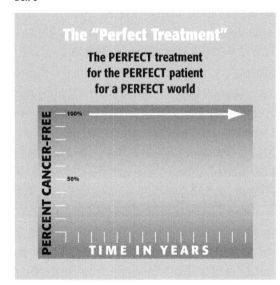

The "Perfect Treatment"

The PERFECT treatment for the PERFECT patient for a PERFECT world

Figure 1

The graph in Figure 1 of the "Perfect Treatment" describes a treatment that is a 100% effective, the so-called "magic bullet." It's important to understand as a concept in order to compare that perfect graph to graphs showing the actual percentages of patients that are treated successfully over time, measured in years after therapy. When the curve of the treatment flattens or plateaus on the graph, this indicates those patients have been treated successfully and the cancer eradicated.

But in reality, we have studies, for example, following patients for many years after radical surgery and their curves never flatten or plateau. The graphs in Figure 2 reflect one early Stanford study done before the PSA era. Each of the curves in those graphs continues to fall, indicating that patients' treatments were continuing to fail over time. It's not very encouraging when measuring survival and failures, because it also indicates that people are dying from prostate cancer, a fact which is sometimes glossed over in the literature. The graphs also indicate that patients who showed no clinical local failure did better than patients who failed clinically – again, this study was done before patients were monitored with the PSA assay.

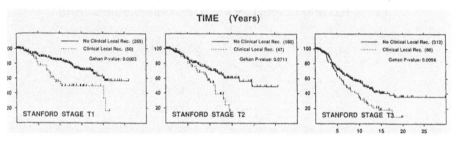

Figure 2: Disease-specific survival following primary definitive treatment, stratified by Stages T1-T3 (Kaplan, J Urol, 147, 1992)

Many patients who have surgery for their prostate cancer are told by their physicians after the operation, "We got it all out." But a number of studies have shown that is very often the case. The falling curve of the graph in Figure 3 shows that even with those cases where all the cancer was apparently removed, the results are not encouraging. And in cases where all the cancer was not removed, meaning the margins were positive for cancer or there was seminal vesicle involvement or perineural invasion, the results are even worse. Many patients are surprised because they think if they go through the rigors of surgery and have their prostates removed that they won't have to worry about prostate cancer anymore. They think that perhaps they will only have to cope with the side effects of the operation, and that their cancer will never return.

But that is really not the case. In fact, in a study done at Johns Hopkins, breaking down the PSA values of patients at the time of surgery, those with PSAs of 3 or 4 fare the best, but surgical patients with PSAs of 10 to 20 are failing at a high rate (see Figure 4). This is a long-term surgical study from Johns Hopkins, with 14 years follow-up, using PSA analysis. And if we look at patients categorized by Gleason scores (Figure 5), even those with a Gleason grade of 7 are failing in large numbers. Many men think "I have an aggressive cancer, I better get it out of me," but the graph shows that most of them are not faring well with that strategy. In fact, if you have a more aggressive cancer, the data shows that the likelihood of surviving for 10 years is low, only about 25%.

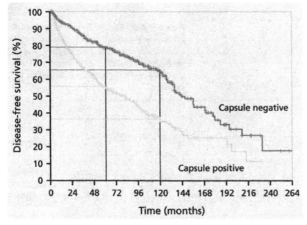

Figure 3: Recurrence after Prostatectomy: Outcomes when cancer has or has not been removed as indicated by capsular involvement (Sterenchock, based on Center for Prostate Disease Database, Urology Times, 2004)

This surgical data is distressing because these are patients who had positive margins and negative margins, but over time most of them are failing as indicated by the linear fall-off of the graph. Radical surgery continues failing at 5 and 10 and 15 years.

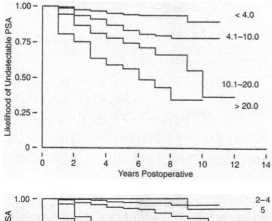

Figure 4 : Likelihood of biochemical failure (rising PSA) by pre-operative serum PSA. *The Oncologist, 8, 2003 (Johns Hopkins)*

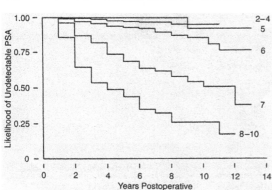

Figure 5: Likelihood of biochemical failure (rising PSA) by pre-operative biopsy Gleason score. *The Oncologist, 8, 2003 (Johns Hopkins)*

The graph in Figure 6 below shows biochemical disease-free outcome for a radical prostatectomy (Katz et al), a three-dimensional conformal radiation therapy (Bonin et al), and a permanent prostate brachytherapy (Merrick et al) series stratified by the presence of perineural invasion (PNI).

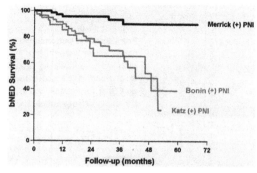

Figure 6: Biochemical disease-free outcome for a radical prostatectomy, three-dimensional conformal radiation therapy, and a permanent prostate brachytherapy series stratified by the presence of perineural invasion.

Does conventional external beam radiation (EBRT) do any better? The answer is not really. A study from Fox Chase showed that patients with favorable risk features have about a 78% survival rate at 10 years, but patients with unfavorable risk features, such as high PSAs, are failing at a high rate, as indicated by the falling curves in the Figure 7.

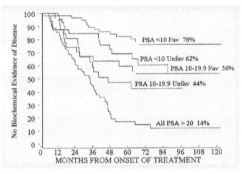

Figure 7: Recurrence after radiation. Long-term 3D-CRT Data. Hanks, IJROBP, Vol 54, 2002 (Fox Chase).

So it's not just surgery that carries a high risk of relapse. Another study from Brigham with 3D-Conformal Radiation Therapy, using a higher dose than conventional external beam radiation, breaks it down into low, intermediate and high risk groups, with the same falling curves indicating a high failure rate for those patients at higher risk (See Figure 8).

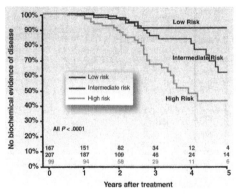

Figure 8: External radiation results stratified by risk groups.

DART: Dynamic Targeting and Accuracy

The Right Place! The Right Dose! The Right Time!

IS LOCALLY ADVANCED HIGH RISK CANCER INCURABLE?
ABSOLUTELY NOT!

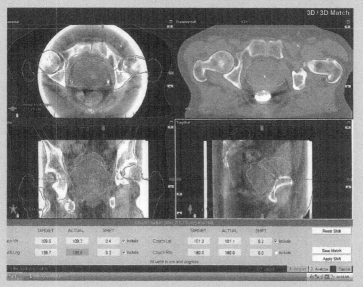

Treating Abdominal or Para-Aortic Nodes Utilizing DART

DART is the ultimate evolution and revolution of IMRT, utilizing all of the most sophisticated imaging and diagnostic modalities. DART involves the modulation of both prescription dose and target delivery based on the actual daily delivered dose, taking into account organ motion, even the motion caused by breathing. This allows for inter/intra fraction verification. At our institution, IMRT in and of itself has become obsolete and we have moved on to the point where with DART we can hit a moving target the size of dot, which is called a voxel, that is 1 cubic millimeter. This enables us to treat patients, both primary and salvage, with an astonishing accuracy that goes well beyond our capabilities even ten years ago.

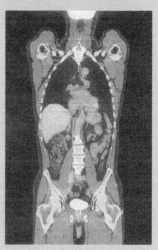

18F-FDG Fluoride PET/CT.
Note: right pelvic lymphadenopathy.

DART: The Most Sophisticated Equipment Anywhere

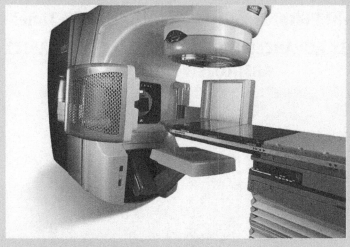

Pictured here is the advanced linear accelerator that delivers precisely targeted beamlets of radiation.

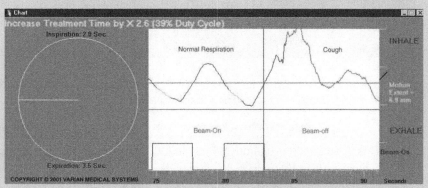

DART and Respiratory Gating – allows for adjustments to take into account a patient's respiration during treatment.

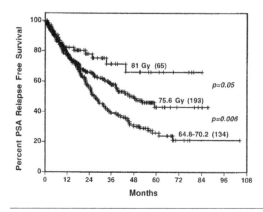

Figure 9: IMRT, Zelefsky et al.– Yes, Dose Matters!

Better results are now being obtained with the more advanced form of external radiation known as Intensity Modulated Radiation Therapy (IMRT). The first study from Memorial Sloan-Kettering Medical Center showed the dose of radiation has been pushed higher than with other forms of external radiation therapy, including 3-Dimensional Conformal Radiation Therapy (3D-CRT) (Zelefsky et al, J of Urol, 166, 2001). These researchers also stratified their results by risk groups (see graphs below, Figures 9 and 10). We know that there is a better cancer-killing response with higher doses. In other words, higher doses show greater success at eradicating the cancer. We expect these results to continue to improve because we are now able to zero in on the target more effectively. We can identify where the cancer is to treat both the prostate and surrounding areas that are affected.

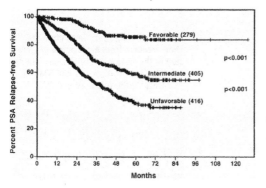

Figure 10: *IMRT, Zelefsky et al.– Yes, Dose Matters*

At our institution, we offer Dynamic Adaptive Radiotherapy (DART), utilizing all of the modalities associated with the most advanced form of IMRT, known as Image-Guided Intensity Modulated Radiation Therapy (IG-IMRT). This new generation of DART technology is used in conjunction with state of the art 3-D Color-Flow Power Doppler Ultrasound, Helical CT Imaging, Respiratory Gating, Theraseed® Palladium-103 Brachytherapy, and Biological Adaptive Fusion capabilities.

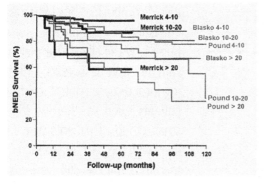

Figure 11: Biochemical disease free survival (bNED) for prostatectomy *(Pound et al)* and brachytherapy published studies *(Blasko et al, Merrick et al)*, with patients stratified by pretreatment PSA level *(J of Brachy Int., Vol. 17, July-Sept. 2001, 193).*

Better outcomes are being achieved with brachytherapy (seed implants) even when utilized as a monotherapy, without supplemental external radiation. The graphs in Figures 11 and 12 compare the results obtained by Dr. John Blasko's brachytherapy group in Seattle and the results reported by Dr. Gregory Merrick's brachytherapy group in Virginia with the results obtained by surgery at Johns Hopkins (Pound et al). The patients were stratified by PSA and Gleason scores. While the surgical curves continue to fall in both of these graphs, the brachytherapy curves flatten or plateau into straight lines, indicating fewer failures with each risk group.

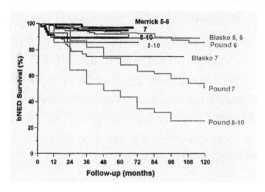

Figure 12: Biochemical disease-free survival (bNED) for prostatectomy (Pound et al) and brachytherapy published studies (Blasko et al, Merrick et al) with patients stratified by Gleason scores of at least 5 (J of Brachy Int., Vol. 17, July-Sept. 2001, 193).

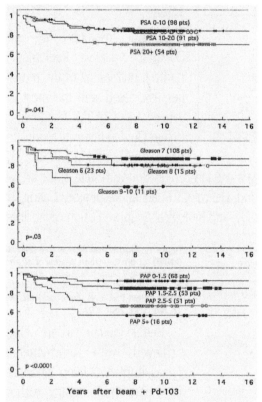

Figures 13, 14 and 15: These three graphs show freedom from biochemical progression of the disease out to 16 years stratified by PSA, Gleason score and PAP (Dattoli, et al, J.Oncol. 2010, Article ID 471375).

Figures 13, 14 and 15 show our own published series for higher risk patients, most of whom had Stage T3 disease, PSA values greater than 15 and Gleason scores of 7 to 10. The success rate was 82% at 16 years. These patients were treated with a protocol combining brachytherapy and external radiation. After some bumps, we finally had a plateau with the curve at six years, indicating local disease control for most patients. Even so, there is still a small group of patients who fail even with the best treatment, and therefore, there is still some reason for concern about recurrence. The patients who experience treatment failure probably had cancer outside the prostate before being treated, but those patients whose cancer was confined show a long and consistent success rate.

What Are The Treatment Options If Surgery Fails?

In men who show a measurable PSA after surgery (as mentioned earlier, often defined by a PSA nadir of 0.2 or a rising trend), the likelihood is that some cancer was left at the margins of the prostate in the surgical bed or that some cancer may have spread to other areas of the body, even though it may not have been previously detected by lymph node dissection or by bone scans. In these cases, further surgery is not advisable, whether robotic or open.

My cancer has returned following primary treatment. What do I do now?
An Overview of Potential Strategies

INITIAL TREATMENT	SALVAGE REGIME
Prostatectomy	EBRT preferably more advanced DART IMRT +/-ADT
EBRT	Salvage Brachytherapy +/- ADT, Cryosurgery, HIFU, Biothermy, Prostatectomy
Brachytherapy	Salvage Brachytherapy +/- IMRT +/- ADT Cryosurgery, HIFU, Biothermy, Prostatectomy

The common forms of salvage therapy for patients who are at risk for failure after surgery are radiation therapy and hormonal therapy. Many patients are clinically understaged and are found to have positive surgical margins, cancer beyond the gland and outside the surgical field, or to have extracapsular extension or seminal vesicle involvement either at the time of surgery or pathologically.

Some of these patients may opt for Active Surveillance (AS) to see if their PSA starts rising before they decide to embark on another course of therapy. Patients who opt for AS after local failure with surgery must be monitored very carefully. Waiting means being prepared to treat specific symptoms of the disease with radiation and/or hormonal therapies if and when it becomes necessary to do so.

What are the Problems with Active Surveillance?

Supportive data for this approach was based on older flawed European studies, primarily because the patients were given hormonal therapy which undermined the data.

➤ 2003 UCSF/CAPSURE trial (watchful waiting Vs prostatectomy >10,000 patients) closed after only 5 years due to adverse findings, i.e. 72% of watchful waiting patients required Androgen deprivation

➤ 2006 Medicare SEER data (U.S. study of men ages 65-80) found very statistically significant benefit to treatment (radiation or surgery)

➤ 2008 Lancet Oncology Study, found prostate cancer mortality in the U.S. to improve over 4-fold since 1994 when compared to men in the U.K. (while the mortality declined and was sustained in U.S. patients aged 75 and older.

➤ 2010 European study (follow up 14 years) demonstrated 27% decrease in mortality with screening and treatment compared to the non screening group (Hugosson J, et al, Lancet, August 2010, 725-732)

Instead of waiting for the PSA to signal a recurrence of cancer, many doctors encourage post-surgical patients to begin a course of radiation therapy in the hope of avoiding problems later. This is referred to as *adjuvant radiation therapy.* Radiation is delivered to the prostatic region in the hope that it will destroy any cancer that may remain there. External radiation following surgery has been shown to reduce the risk of biochemical relapse (rising PSA) by approximately 30% (as evidenced by the fact that about 30% of men show an undetectable PSA after salvage radiation). To reduce the risk of complications, doctors usually allow surgical patients to recover for 3 to 6 months before starting radiation therapy.

Adjuvant Radiation Matters: SWOG 8794– Patterns of failure associated with high-risk prostate cancer.

This study showed that there was a dramatic improvement in results with patients treated with adjuvant radiation immediately after surgery versus those patients who waited to fail with rising PSA. This study also showed that most of the lymph node involvement was in the true pelvis and upper pelvis. This suggests treating the higher pelvic region to be a benefit.

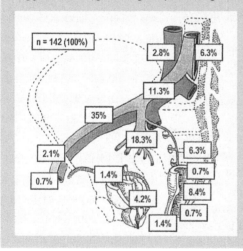

Anatomic distribution of sentinel nodes (SN) as detected by single photon emission computed tomographic imaging in 25 patients. *Sentinel Node-based IMRT for Prostate Cancer Int J. Rad Onc, Vol 67, No 2, 347-355*

External radiation is the most common salvage treatment for presumed local failure after surgery, while hormonal therapy is most often prescribed in cases of distant failure and evidence of metastatic disease. Some doctors favor using hormonal therapy after surgery as soon as there is any evidence of recurrence. The rationale is that hormones may slow the progress of the disease for some time.

Hormonal therapy is not curative, but hormones do interrupt the spread of the disease temporarily. For some men, this knowledge may be enough to prompt them to try some form of hormonal intervention early on. Other patients may prefer to wait. Recent data, however, suggest that early hormonal intervention is superior to delayed treatment. For recurrence, we use radiation combined with a limited course of hormones for salvage therapy.

Depending on the particular hormone or combination of hormones that are prescribed, many men experience some side effects such as erectile dysfunction, loss of sexual desire (libido), breast enlargement, hot flashes, nausea, diarrhea, liver enzyme elevation, muscle weakness, joint aches or pains, and bone fragility (loss of bone integrity). Depending on the type of hormone prescribed, there are also a number of medications and treatment options which can be used to minimize or ameliorate these side effects. For more information on this subject, readers are referred to the Prostate Cancer Essentials booklet, *Hormonal Therapy for Prostate Cancer: The Benefits and Risks.*

Outcomes With Salvage Radiation Following Prostatectomy

As noted, after failed prostatectomy, radiation may be a viable option. Most surgeons suggest that if a patient has a rising PSA after surgery, he should have radiation. One study from Duke reported about a 30% to 40% salvage or rescue rate (Anscher, IJROBP, Vol. 48, 2000—see Figure 14). Those results were not very encouraging.

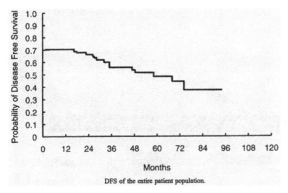

DFS of the entire patient population.

Figure 14: Anscher et al, Duke.

When we see patients with rising PSAs after surgery, we have to figure out if we are going to treat the prostate region because we believe that is where the cancer is. We want to know if the patient's Gleason score was less than or equal to 7, whether or not there was seminal vesicle invasion at the time of surgery, whether or not the lymph nodes were involved, how long after surgery his PSA started rising, and what the PSA velocity and doubling time are—all of these can help us to predict whether the disease is still localized or has metastasized.

With patients who have a rising PSA after surgery, we make every effort to determine whether local or distant failure is indicated. We will do a bone scan and a number of other tests to determine if the cancer is aggressive and may have metastasized. We also test bone density because hormonal agents may affect bone integrity. Some of the agents that we use to enhance bone strength also have an anti-cancer effect. We like to look at other things beyond the PSA, including Ploidy status using DNA histograms and other histochemical stains to determine how aggressive the cancer is. Nano-particle testing is also helpful in this regard, as is 18F Flouride PET/CT.

Unlike many other treatment centers, we aggressively treat not only locally advanced recurrent patients, but those with distant metastases as well. Patients with distant metastases are candidates for salvage treatment with radiation because we use multiple strategies for recurrence with those patients that may include DART, but also Samarium-153-EDTMP (Quadramet®), hormones and injectable biphosphonates, so they are not considered just palliative care patients who are minimally treated to alleviate side effects. We give these patients not only an aggressive workup to determine the extent of disease, but we plan on aggressively treating ALL KNOWN SITES OF DISEASE, which will include bones and lymph nodes in many patients. This is not to say that we are able to cure these patients, but by treating all the malignant sites we can identify, these patients are living longer with a better quality of life; so it is a far better method of controlling their disease as much as possible.

What Factors Are Important With Salvage Radiation?

It appears that a low PSA before starting treatment after surgery is an important factor, as is the dose of radiation delivered. The higher the dose the more likely it is that the cancer will be eradicated.

Salvage Radiotherapy for PSA-Only Recurrence Following Radical Prostatectomy

AUTHOR	PRE-SALVAGE PSA	DISEASE-FREE OUTCOME AT 5 YRS
Wu et al	>2.5	8%
Forman et all	>2.0	33%
	<2.0	59%
Stephenson et al	>2.0	15%
	≤2.0	52%
Zelefsky et all	>1.0	17%
	<1.0	74%

Scionti, AUA, 2004

Clinical and Pathological Predictors in Patients with PSA Failure after Radical Prostatectomy

DISTANT METASTASIS (GLEASON ≥7)	LOCAL RECURRENCE (GLEASON <7)
• Seminal vesicle invasion	• No seminal vesicle invasion
• Positive pelvic lymph nodes	• Negative pelvic lymph nodes
• PSA detectable less than 1 year after surgery	• PSA detectable more than 1 year after surgery
• PSA velocity greater than 0.75 ng/ml	• PSA velocity less than 0.75 ng/ml
• Doubling time less than 6 months	• Doubling time greater than 6 months

Study by Scattoni et al, Amer J Urol Rev, 2004

Perhaps the biggest problem after surgery is the condition of the tissue. As mentioned earlier, radiation works best in an oxygenated field. It depends on oxygen molecules to create free radicals to kill the cancer cells. After prostatectomy, the prostate bed is for the most part devascularized scar tissue which is poorly oxygenated. In addition, conventional salvage radiation doses are sub-optimal since both the rectum and bladder now occupy the target region. The solution to this post-surgical situation is to increase radiation doses using highly sophisticated radiation modalities (preferably DART) and to combine radiation with hormones to exploit the synergistic supra-additive effects (e.g. 1+1=3 or 4)

The time to PSA relapse is also an important consideration, whether it began to rise two months or ten years after treatment. Other factors include the original Gleason grade and whether or not there was seminal vesicle invasion.

Adjuvant versus Salvage Radiation after Prostatectomy

Historical Perspective Derived from Evidence-based Data

After surgery, if the PSA rises to a certain point, patients may be treated with radiation and/or hormonal therapy. In that case, the radiation is a salvage therapy (SRT), which attempts to cure patients after surgery has failed. Adjuvant radiation therapy (ART) is planned in advance for surgical patients identified as having adverse features within the postoperative pathological specimens. It is planned that these patients will receive post-operative radiation 8 to 12 weeks after they have surgery. Surveys show that only 7% to 13% of urologists refer patients for adjuvant radiation and/or hormonal therapy, so those options are underutilized.

Here we will summarize the results of a number of studies that investigated adjuvant and salvage radiation therapy, as well as hormonal therapy. One NCI trial reported that after surgery when the PSA reached 0.21 to 0.5, 48% of patients who received salvage radiation survived at 6 years. The percentage of patients surviving fell to only 8% when the PSA rose to 1.51. So the earlier patients are treated after the PSA begins to rise post-surgery the better the outcome with salvage radiation. What the study shows, summarized below, is how even that incremental rise in PSA impacts the biochemical freedom of progression of disease and overall survival after salvage radiation.

NCI Prostate Cancer SPORE Study

Predicting Outcomes of Salvage Radiation

Multi-institutional, 1,540 consecutive pT3 patients

➤ Endpoint PSA >0.2 ng/ml Following RP

Results at 6 years

Overall 6 year biochemical free progression = 32%

48% when post-op PSA: 0.21–0.5

40% when post-op PSA: 0.51–1.0

28% when post-op PSA: 1.01–1.5

18% when post-op PSA: > 1.51

➤ Side effects: acute RTOG 3-4 toxicity and late Grade 3 < 4%

➤ Shortcoming: low RT dose, 70 Gy

Conclusion: Benefit of Salvage Radiation Inversely Correlated to PSA Level

Stephenson et al, J Clin Onc, 25, 2055-61, 2007

Another study (SWOG 87-94) published in 2009 compared patients who were given adjuvant radiation 8 to 12 months after surgery with patients who received salvage radiation and hormones later after their PSA began to rise following surgery. These researchers reported that at 12.7 years follow-up the patients who received adjuvant radiation had a 59% survival rate, while patients who received salvage radiation therapy had a 48% survival rate. That shows that adjuvant radiation really has a statistically significant impact, as summarized below.

Between the two groups of patients there was no statistical difference with side effects involving urination, bowels and erectile function. This finding is consistent with numerous other past and ongoing studies. In other words, a man's quality of life after having surgery will not be altered by subsequent radiation therapy. Quality of life is not affected by postsurgical adjuvant or salvage radiation.

Supportive Data for Postsurgical Adjuvant Radiation Therapy (ART)

SWOG 87-94: (Randomized Clinical Trial – Long Term Follow-up)

➤ Adjuvant radiation therapy for pT3 NoMo prostate cancer
➤ Endpoint overall survival and metastasis-free survival
   425 consecutive patients
   Median follow-up 12.7 years

	MEDIAN OVERALL SURVIVAL	METASTASIS-FREE SURVIVAL
214 patients (adjuvant RT, 60-64Gy)	59%	93/214
211 patients (observation –	48%	114/211
salvage RT upon failure + ADT)	p = 0.023	p = 0.034

Quality of Life: No statistical difference between the two groups with urination/bowels/erectile function

NOTE: Doses 60-64Gy to "pelvic fossa," low by contemporary standards.

Thompson et al, J Urology: Vol 181, 956-62, 2009

With this next study published in 2012, researchers followed one group of post-surgical patients who received radiation after their PSA rose to 0.2, and another group of postsurgical patients who were given radiation post-operatively (adjuvant). The results at 10 years were 61.% biochemical progression-free survival for the patients who received post-operative radiation versus 39.4% of patients who watched and waited until their PSA was rising before being treated with radiation. The 0.001 p value indicates the difference in outcomes was statistically significant.

Supportive data for Adjuvant Radiation Therapy (ART)
EORTC 22911:
Randomized 1,005 consecutive patients with pT3 disease, following RP
   Arm A—"Wait and see": (initiate post-op RT when PSA > 0.2)
   Arm B—adjuvant post-op RT (8 weeks median 64Gy, pre-3D-IMRT era)
   Median follow-up 10.6 years.

Results
10 year biochemical progression-free survival:
   Arm A—39.4%
   Arm B—61.8%
   P = < 0.001

Arm B: Also improved clinical progression-free survival; (p = 0.009), reduced local-regional failure (p = 0.005).

Overall survival did not reach statistical significance (p = 0.04)

NOTE: Nearly 50% of relapsing patients in the observation group received deferred radiation, yet the Arm B group had an advantage with biochemical disease free survival (the overall survival would likely have reached significance had this study continued).

Grade III toxicity 4.2% vs 2.6% (p=0.052) Arm B

Bolla et al, Lancet 380: 2018-27, 2012

Another important study was done in Milan, Italy, and it tested adjuvant radiation combined with hormonal therapy versus hormonal therapy alone for postsurgical patients. The combined treatments of radiation and hormones are called a multi-modal approach. This trial was really asking the question does radiation have an impact.

95% and 86% of patients who received the radiation and hormones survived at 5 and 10 years respectively while 88% and 70% of patients who received hormones alone survived at 5 and 10 years respectively. Now these were patients who had positive lymph nodes either after surgery, and again, the outcomes are statistically significant at 10 years, with a 16% difference and patients who had the radiation and hormones having better cancer specific survival.

Milan Matched Analysis Trial

Supportive data for both Post-op Radiation Therapy and ADT (multi-modal)

Combination of Adjuvant Hormonal Therapy and Post-op Radiation Therapy prolongs survival in patients having pT2-4 pN1 prostate cancer:

Results of matched analysis

367 consecutive patients

      Group I—117 pT2-4 pN1 → ADT + RT (3DCRT, median 6840)

      Group II—247 pT2-4 pN1 → ADT alone

Median follow-up 100.8 months

Cancer Specific Survival

	5 YEARS	10 YEARS
Group I (post-op ADT + RT)	95%	86%
Group II (post-op ADT alone)	88%	70%
	p = < 0.004	

Briganti et al, European Urol, 59: 832-40, 2011) (Milan)

The M.D. Anderson RTOG 85-31study published in 2005 and summarized below followed patients with lymph node disease who either had a radical prostatectomy (RP) or their prostates were intact upon presentation. They were treated with a multi-modal approach. With two groups of patients, 488 received Adjuvant Radiation Therapy (ART) and hormones while 489 received radiation and hormones only after their PSA rose above 0.2. The first group fared better with surgery, radiation and hormones in terms of absolute survival, disease free survival, biochemical disease free survival, and even with patients having Gleason 7 to 10 scores.

RTOG 85-31

Clinical state pT3 pN1 disease treated with RT or RP + adjuvant vs delayed. In the RTOG 85-31 trial, patients received, neo-adjuvant 2 month ADT + during RT for bulky tumors resulting in statistical improvement in all end points (including Absolute Survival though only in Gleason scores ≤ 6)

977 randomized patients

Arm I 488 patients – adjuvant ADT (begin final week of RT, then indefinitely)

if RT—pelvic RT, 44-50Gy and 20-25Gy prostate boost

if RP—prostate bed treated to 60-65Gy

Arm II 489 patients—observation following RP/RT, ADT when loco-regional progression/distant mets or PSA ≥ 1.5

Results: Kaplan-Meier + Multivariate Cox Proportional hazard regression

Patients in Arm I benefited at 10 years vs Arm II

Absolute survival—48% vs 36% (p < 0.03)

Disease free survival—38% vs 23% (p = 0.014)

Biochemical disease survival—31% vs 9% (p < 0.0001)

Gleason 7-10 survival—40% vs 30% (p = 0.0039)

Pilepich et al, Int J Rad Onc, Vol 61, No 5, 1285-90, 2005

We are cautious about using hormonal therapy at our center because hormones do have some downsides with significant side effects, but this study and others have demonstrated that hormones can have significant advantages when combined with radiation.

Another study from the Fox Chase Cancer Center followed high-risk patients with Gleason scores 8-10 treated by pelvic radiation and hormonal therapy before and during radiation therapy, or by pelvic radiation combined with hormonal therapy (LH-RH) that continued 2 years after treatment. That study showed the patients who received post-radiation hormones for 2 years had an 81% survival rate versus 70% for those patients whose hormonal therapy ended immediately after radiation therapy (*Hanks et al, J Clin Onc, 21, 3972-8, 2003*). As noted, we are not overly enthusiastic about hormones, especially in the long term, but with the preponderance of data from various studies, we are obligated to offer hormonal therapy to patients, explaining the possible benefits and risks they can expect with hormones.

It should be noted that RTOG 92-02 reported similar survival rates with Gleason 8-10 patients, while the EORTC 22911 study showed that all Gleason scores benefited with respect to all endpoints except Overall Survival. The study showed prolonged biochemical disease-free survival and cancer specific survival. Gleason scores 8-10 appeared to benefit most, though not statistically.

Another evidence-based study, RTOG 96-01, showed the advantage of two years of hormonal therapy after surgery using 150 mg of Casodex. 57% of patients who received hormones showed no biochemical progression versus 40% who received a placebo instead of hormonal therapy. These two groups of patients, arms 1 and 2, were followed a median of 7.1 years. Patients with Gleason scores 8 to 10 benefited the most. Some patients did have problems with gynecomastia, breast enlargement due to the Casodex. We do have various ways to deal with the gynecomastia problem. The researchers suggested a follow up study using a lower dose of that hormonal agent to 50 mg to see if that would alter the results. A related question now being studied is if the use of hormones can be reduced if the radiation dose is increased.

RTOG 96-01

Randomized, multi-center trial comparing post-op salvage RT and 150mg Casodex for 2 years to post-op salvage RT and placebo in men with pT_{2-3} N1 prostate cancer who have an elevated PSA after RP.

Preliminary results: (12/13/10)
> Median follow-up 7.1 years with 771 eligible patients
> Freedom from biochemical progression
> Arm 1—57% in EBRT + Casodex
> Arm 2—40% in EBRT + Placebo
> $p = < 0.003$

Benefits greatest with Gleason 8-10 patients: Gynecomastia problematic in the Casodex Arm 1 group. Question: would 50 mg Casodex demonstrate same impact?

Ambrowitz et al, Semin Rad Onc 18: 15-22, 2008

Finally, the EORTC 22863 study looked at patients with intact prostates, those who had not had surgery but had high risk features, such as Gleason scores 8 to 10. One group of patients was treated with pelvic radiation and given hormonal therapy in the form of an LH-RH agonist, while a second group of patients received pelvic radiation alone. They did find a statistically significant benefit with hormones. As you can see in the summary below, those who received hormonal therapy fared better in terms of 10-year overall survival and cancer specific survival than those patients who were not given hormones. We would be reluctant to use hormones for three years because of the risk of side effects problems. We would instead use a far more abbreviated hormonal regime (6 to 13 months). Hormones can exacerbate cardiovascular problems. Interestingly, this study found no cardiac incidents over a follow up period of 10 years.

So it appears there is a benefit using radiation (with or without hormones) with lymph node positive patients, but what about side effects? No trial using adjuvant radiation therapy and/or salvage radiation therapy has demonstrated a statistically significant detriment to erectile function compared to radical prostatectomy alone. Nor has any ART or SRT trial demonstrated statistically significant bowel or bladder dysfunction without resolution at 2 to 5 years compared to baseline scores. *In fact, both ART and SRT trials are associated with < 1% radiation-related morbidities.* So the risk of side effects is remarkably low with radiation, not impacting what would otherwise be expected (quite contrary to what patients are often told).

EORTC 22863
High-Risk, Intact Locally Advanced Prostate Cancer
Stage T$_3$/T$_4$ or high-grade Gleason 8-10

415 consecutive patients randomized

    Group A—Pelvic RT alone (208)

    Group B—Pelvic RT + LH-RH agonist for 3 years (207)

Median follow-up 10 years

	GROUP A		GROUP B
10 year overall survival	47%	vs	39.8% (p = 0.0004)
Cancer specific survival	30.4%	vs	10.3%

No significant adverse cardiac events.

Bolla et al, Lancet Oncol: 11: 1066-1073, 2010

And yet, even with the results of these major trials showing the benefits of radiation for surgery patients, only about 10% of urologists send their surgical patients for radiation. This is especially distressing when we consider the growing body of evidence supporting early postsurgical intervention with radiation.

Most studies suggest that salvage patients after surgery have approximately ten times the disease burden compared to patients treated with adjuvant radiation, and multiple prospective randomized trials have demonstrated a benefit for Adjuvant Radiation over Salvage Radiation. These comparison studies looked at Salvage Radiation with low PSA and especially Gleason scores 8 to10, seminal vesicle involvement, and positive margins (RTOG 7506; 8531, SWOG 8794; EORTC 29111). The multi-modal approach appears superior, increasing overall survival (RTOG 9202, RTOG 9601, EORTC 22863).

Salvage Radiation appears to be appropriate for patients who have the highest chance of having local regional disease:

➤ PSA doubling time > 12 months   ➤ Interval to PSA failure ≥ 3 years

➤ Positive surgical margins   ➤ Gleason 7 or lower

So the take-home message for patients who have had surgery is don't wait too long to begin Salvage Radiation. As a patient, you should be proactive with your urologist or oncologist, because many of them don't pay attention to the fact that if your PSA rises above 2.0, you're very unlikely to benefit from radiation or hormone or anything else. That number has been whittled down over the years, so it's now really between 0.2 and 0.6–after that the results fall off for patients having successful outcomes.

Various studies are underway, but preliminary data suggests significant benefit to Adjuvant RT while the benefit of Salvage RT is inversely correlated to serum PSA at time of RT. Patients with PSA values higher than 0.4 are less likely to be cured by Salvage RT. While there is still some uncertainty about Adjuvant versus Salvage radiation after surgery, the data shows that salvage is viable for most patients, but they have to keep a very close eye on the PSA to catch it rising early enough to get better results. That's very important to understand because it really is a matter of survival.

Doctors who see the rising PSA after surgery will often just monitor their patients with active surveillance (watchful waiting), but that concept really shouldn't apply to postsurgical patients. It applies to newly diagnosed patients who have very low risk cancer, not to high-risk postsurgical patients. In any case, active surveillance doesn't mean just having your PSA checked once a year, actually means biannually if not quarterly, as well as being biopsied at least once a year and having the PCA3 urine test. It also means undergoing periodical (annual or biannual) advanced imaging studies including but not limited to multi-parametric MRIs and 3D Color-Flow Doppler Ultrasound, which we use at the Dattoli Cancer Center.

What Are The Risks Of Side Effects After Salvage IMRT?

The bladder, urethra, rectum, and sexual function can all be affected with radiation. We use RTOG analysis for scoring the severity of symptoms. Fortunately we have alpha-blockers that can help in cases of an agitated prostate or bladder. For managing urinary symptoms, we may prescribe alpha-blockers such as Uroxatrol® (Alfuzosin), Flomax® (Tamsulosin), Rapaflo, Hytrin or Cardura. These medications relax the prostate and bladder and have been very helpful with our patients. We also recommend over-the-counter anti-inflammatory remedies and supplements.

A study from Baylor University Medical Center has shown that when using radiation as salvage therapy with doses of 75 Gy and higher with IMRT that the patients have much less bladder or rectal toxicity when compared to conventional radiation or 3D-CRT. IMRT also had no adverse effect on sexual function. The study demonstrated that if a patient is potent after nerve-sparing surgery, he will be potent after IMRT. This is because with IMRT and DART, we can avoid irradiating the penile bulb and crus, which are beneath the prostate and appear to be essential to normal sexual function. While using DART at higher doses, we're finding far less toxicity than with other forms of external radiation for post-surgical patients with rising PSAs. We prescribe prophylactic low dose Viagra, Cialis, or Levitra protocols during and after treatment.

When Is Hormonal Therapy Combined With Salvage Radiation?

We have a compilation of recent studies, including RTOG, that suggest the use of hormonal therapy is beneficial when combined with salvage radiation. With patients having prostate cancer with high risk features (high PSA, high Gleason score), we found these patients to have benefited in terms of disease-free survival and even overall survival. The common thread in all these studies is that at some point the radiation was given simultaneously with hormonal therapy. If a patient fails prostatectomy because of the fact that he has a high Gleason score, indicating a more aggressive cancer, there may be a benefit to using hormonal therapy in his case just as we do those patients who receive radiation as a primary treatment.

A Stanford University Medical Center study showed results with 10 years actuarial follow up with 56.8% success rate with radiation plus hormones versus 31.2%

with radiation alone (King et al., Int J Rad Onc, Vol.59, No.2, 2004, pp 341-347). Numerous other studies have shown the advantage of combining radiation with hormones: EORTC (Bolla), RTOG 94-13, RTOG 92-02, RTOG 85-13, RTOG 86-10, and Messing, NEJM, Vol. 341, 1999.

What Are The Treatment Options If External Radiation Fails?

We have learned that prostate cancer cells are amazingly adaptable—in fact, they can quickly become resistant to external radiation, making it less effective. That fact underscores our choice of combined radiation therapy whenever possible. We have found that by delivering approximately half the "tumor-cidal" (killing) dose of radiation through an external process and implanting the other half through brachytherapy intensifies the response, giving higher cure rates with lower side effects. Cancers don't like change! By combining different forms of radiation, we increase the odds for success.

In fact, cross specialty studies looking at breast cancer, colorectal cancer, head and neck cancers, etc. *all* demonstrate an increasing survival rate when a combination of therapies is used.

We don't subscribe to the philosophy that if a patient has had previous radiation therapy, he is no longer a candidate for further radiation, since most of these failures are due to the failure of the physician in not delivering a proper dose and areas of tissue untreated inadequately, etc. So we are often able to re-treat with radiation after reviewing the dosimetry of the previous treatment.

Patients experiencing recurrence following single modality radiation are often eligible for additional treatment using a different form of radiation. For instance, the man who had EBRT alone may benefit from a small dose of DART followed immediately by seed implant (depending on the location of the active cancer cells).

Patients who are not cured by any of the various forms of external radiation therapy *(external beam, etc. with or without brachytherapy, or brachytherapy alone)* have various options for salvage therapy, including even radical surgery. The operation to remove the prostate is more difficult after radiation, and some doctors do not recommend salvage prostatectomy because of their own limited experience. They will inform the patient that the risk of complications is high, while the likelihood of cure is relatively low. Nonetheless, salvage prostatectomy remains an option in experienced surgical hands. However, we do not recommend salvage surgery, open or robotic, because in our opinion that approach would be useless as the spread of cancer is typically not only in the gland but also outside the prostate, so that removing the gland would not solve the problem.

One group at Baylor in Texas was led by Dr. Peter Scardino who is currently at Memorial Sloan-Kettering. That group found that there was approximately a 50% survival rate with salvage surgery; however, there was also a 50% rate of incontinence. Salvage surgery remains an option, but patients are advised to proceed with caution for the reasons mentioned above.

After primary radiation fails, a second treatment with radiation is often not advised since the first course of radiation did not cure the cancer and the risk of complications is high. However, there is growing interest in treating failed external radiation patients with brachytherapy and/or DART, since seed implant radiation and DART can be focused on the prostate, with less risk of damage to the rectum and surrounding tissue. One recent study reported that as many as 50% of these salvage brachytherapy patients were disease-free at 5 years.

If the recurrent patient had primary radiation, then he has already received a significant dose of radiation which makes additional radiation potentially dangerous. To ensure safety, these men will need the higher doses available only through the sophistication of treatment delivery programs encompassing all the available tools (especially with DART). To maximize the potential of radiation for recurrent patients, we often prescribe hormonal therapy—which creates a positive synergy with radiation resulting in mathematically boosting the effects (1+1 = 3 or 4 or 5, for instance).

Cryosurgery, also called cryoblation, is a primary treatment method that involves the insertion of freezing probes into the prostate to kill cancerous tissue. This technique has also been used as a salvage therapy for locally recurrent prostate cancer after failed radiation, though there is little published data available. One study reported a disease-free survival rate of 74% after two years, but with a very high rate of complications such as incontinence and erectile dysfunction. The incontinence rate may be reduced in experienced hands, but we are not advocates of this approach because of the side effect profile and the paucity of long term data.

When cryosurgery is used as a primary treatment and fails, it can be repeated in many cases, but this is really not an advantage. The idea with a primary treatment is to eradicate the cancer once and for all. Other salvage options after failed cryosurgery include surgery, radiation and hormonal therapy.

Focal cryosurgery (also known as prostate lumpectomy) has also shown some promise as a salvage therapy after radiation when the recurrence is limited to one lobe of the prostate. Researchers at Columbia University Medical Center reported that disease-free survival (DFS) for salvage cryotherapy (SC) at 5 and 10 years follow-up was 63% and 56% respectively (Wenske S, et al, "Salvage cryosurgery of the prostate for failure after primary radiotherapy or cryosurgery" Eur Urol, 2013 Jul; 64 (1):1-7).

A more recent study from the Cleveland Clinic demonstrated modestly favorable results when salvage focal cryosurgery was utilized to treat patients with recurrent cancer after various forms of radiotherapy. With patient follow-up of 1, 3, and 5 years, researchers reported biochemical disease-free survival rates of 95.3%, 72.4%, and 46.5%. Erectile function was retained by 50% of patients, while 5.5% experienced urinary incontinence which required them to wear absorbent pads. Another 6.6% of men suffered from urinary retention after therapy (Li YH, Prostate, 2015 Jan;75(1):1-7).

If a man's PSA after external radiation (or brachytherapy) rises only very slowly over a period of one to three years, then the cancer may still be confined within the prostate. These patients have the most options among those patients whose treatments fail with radiation, including watchful waiting depending on the age and life expectancy of the patient. A number of studies have shown that there are patients with biopsy-detected local recurrence who have survived 10 years or more without experiencing any progression of the disease. However, more aggressive tumors with Gleason scores of 7 to 10 may secrete little PSA, and even a slow PSA rise may be significant with respect to tumor growth and cancer spread.

In addition to salvage treatments like brachytherapy, surgery and cryosurgery, there are also the options of hormonal therapy or even orchiectomy (surgical castration), though the latter is rarely used these days. The same considerations that apply to hormonal therapy after failed surgery apply to hormonal therapy for men with local or distant cancer recurrence after radiation. As discussed earlier, some studies suggest that men treated with a combination of hormones and radiation as their initial treatment have a reduced rate of failure. However, initial radical prostatectomy combined with hormones has not demonstrated a significant benefit.

With the object of shutting down the body's production of testosterone completely, many doctors combine drugs like Lupron® (or Eligard® or Zoladex® or Trelstar®) with Casodex® (or Eulexin®), along with Avodart® and Proscar®, which together provide a total blockage against the male hormones that nourish prostate cancer. For many men, the use of this type of combination hormonal therapy (CHT) to achieve a castration level of testosterone that may slow the progression of the disease is preferable to undergoing orchiectomy, which is a less expensive way to achieve the same end but with permanent and irreversible side effects.

In addition, unlike surgical castration, this form of medical castration is reversible and may be used intermittently. The patients may be on hormones 6 to 12 months, and then completely off hormones until the PSA reaches a predetermined value.

Intermittent hormonal therapy (IHT) allows for recovery of the male bodily functions during the periods when the patient is off hormones.

It should also be noted that patients who have failed novel treatments such as Proton Beam Therapy or Cyberknife need to be carefully evaluated. Regardless of what original primary therapy was used, each case must be assessed individually, as these treatments vary radically in their impact upon the cancerous cells, as well as the healthy cells. In most cases there is some additional treatment that can be utilized. We typically assess the current condition of your prostate and surrounding tissues, recommend the most sensitive diagnostic examinations and laboratory analyses, and then review salvage options with you.

Who Are Candidates For Salvage Brachytherapy After Failed Radiation?

If you've had radiation and your PSA is rising, we may want biopsy confirmation of local recurrence and ideally we would like to wait 2½ to 3 years after initial radiation. We don't always need biopsy confirmation of a local recurrence when implementing salvage brachytherapy. We prefer tissue confirmation, but if the Color-Flow Power Doppler Ultrasound is compelling enough and the dosimetry indicates suboptimal dosing of original implant, then we will not require a biopsy.

If we see a patient with a palpable recurrence through DRE and if the color-flow Doppler shows a possible recurrence, we may be able to avoid a prostatic biopsy, though in some cases we have been using transperineal saturation biopsies. With Color-Flow Power Doppler Ultrasound, we can also limit the number of biopsies on patients who have had radiation before. We don't treat patients who have had RCOG grade III or IV urinary or bowel toxicity.

A study by Dr. David Beyer in Scottsdale, Arizona reported on the issue of salvage brachytherapy and showed a 53% 5-year freedom from relapse using either iodine-125 or palladium-103. Patients who received hormones had a 72% success rate versus 42% for patients who did not receive hormones. With Gleason scores less than or equal to 6, there was an 83% freedom from relapse versus 30% with patients having a Gleason score of 7 or higher (Beyer DC, Oncology, Williston Park, 2004 Feb;18(2):151-8).

Salvage brachytherapy is much more effective before the PSA rises above 10 and with Gleason scores of 6 or less. Dr. Gordon Grado in Scottsdale reported a freedom from relapse rate of 34% at 5 years, but the median PSA for that series was somewhat high at 5.6. Dr. Grado used a urethral and sphincter-sparing technique and reported only a 6% incontinence rate (Grado GL, et al, Salvage brachytherapy for localized prostate cancer after radiotherapy failure; Urology. 1999;53(1):2–10).

With our published data, patients had a median pre-treatment PSA of 10.6, which was high, and more than half had Gleason scores of 8 or higher. Patients who had been treated with iodine were treated with palladium brachytherapy the second time, and vice versa. We also used a minimum of 6 months of hormonal therapy. We found that 55% maintained a PSA less than or equal to 0.2. No patient experienced local disease progression. 2 of 17 patients experienced low-volume stress incontinence. These are compelling results (Dattoli MJ, et al, Neoadjuvant hormone therapy and palladium-103 brachytherapy as salvage for locally recurrent prostate cancer; Proc Am Clin Soc Oncol. 1997;16:1118).

Patients may receive 3 to 6 months of neoadjuvant hormonal therapy (meaning up front, prior to treatment) with a bone integrity agent and/or other agents for patients who have failed external radiation or brachytherapy. As mentioned, with failed brachytherapy patients, we prefer to use a different isotope the second time around. Preferably, the hormones are continued while the patient is receiving radiation. Most patients in this situation receive hormones for a total of approximately 12 months.

Salvage patients receive 9,000 to 10,000 cGy with salvage palladium-103, in contrast to a dose of 12,000 cGy to 13,000 cGy if the patient were receiving primary treatment with palladium brachytherapy. The initial hormonal therapy appears to make the radiation work better at the lower dose. We have had a 50% success rate going out to about 10 years in this population. The good news is that in contemporary studies the incontinence rate has been kept low, at less than 5%. We have minimized the urinary side effects and have had no rectal ulcerations.

Dr. Beyer did a survey of research being done on salvage brachytherapy and found that with as many as 98% of patients, the disease was locally controlled. With carefully selected patients, those having low PSAs, the rate of local control with salvage brachytherapy is almost as great as with patients who had brachytherapy as their primary treatment. A more recent study from the University of Pennsylvania on salvage brachytherapy for recurrence after EBRT reported, "Five and 7-year relapse-free survival, distant metastasis-free survival, and overall survival were 79% and 67%; 93% and 86%; and 94% and 85%, respectively" (Baumann BC, et al, Brachytherapy, 2017 Mar - Apr;16(2):291-298).

What can be done for patients who have had their prostates removed, as well as having salvage external radiation, and now see their PSA is rising again? With these patients there has to be palpable disease in order for an implant to be feasible. After prostatectomy and salvage external radiation, if there is no palpable tumor, those patients would be limited to salvage DART. We look for lymph node and bone metastases using advanced imaging studies such as contrast enhanced MRI and, when indicated, implement salvage therapy.

What Are The Treatment Options If Brachytherapy Fails?

Patients who have had seed implantation without initial success may have the option of being re-seeded. This approach appears to be promising, and as mentioned, typically involves using a different isotope the second time around. If the patient was first implanted with iodine, then palladium might be used as a salvage therapy in the hope that the cancer will be more sensitive to the second isotope. If the first implant was technically mishandled, then a second implant affords the opportunity of correcting misplacements that may have caused underdosing.

As described previously, brachytherapy patients who experience treatment failure also have the salvage options of surgery, cryosurgery, hormonal therapy, and active surveillance. In some cases based on the extent of the disease as determined by workup testing, several months of hormonal therapy may be prescribed to reduce the size of the tumor prior to an attempt at salvage therapy with either cryosurgery or surgery (though we do not recommend surgery for reasons explained earlier).

Meticulous re-staging work-up research is mandatory. We have to know how extensive the disease is. It may be that the PSA value is high, but the disease is still confined to the prostate. Lower pre-salvage PSAs have more favorable outcomes. We want to see patients sooner, before their PSA values reach 5 or 8 or 10.

We use hormonal therapy before, after and during radiation therapy. We also limit the dose of the implant for salvage brachytherapy, which turns out to be effective thanks to enhanced radiosensitivity with hormonal therapy. With hormones, we use an anti-androgen such as Casodex® or Eulexin®, combined with an LHRH agonist such as Zoladex® or Lupron® or Eligard® or Trelstar®. We also use Proscar® and Avodart®.

We use palladium whenever possible because of its steep dose fall off. That means at any distance from the seed, the dose is lower than with any other isotope. That's important with patients who have been previously treated. We don't want to give the patient the same implant that failed previously. Avoiding a hot apex means using urethral sparing techniques in order to avoid implanting the distal or external sphincter, because that patient will run a higher risk of incontinence.

Who is Most Likely to Benefit from Salvage Therapy?

Lower risk patients are most likely to benefit from salvage therapy, those men with low pretreatment PSA values and low pretreatment Gleason scores. Unfortunately, those patients who most require salvage therapy stand to benefit the least. They are men with more aggressive and more advanced disease. An ideal or optimal salvage regime is more appropriate for 1) patients with no seminal vesicle involvement,

2) patients who experience a prolonged disease-free interval of at least a year and preferably 2 years before the PSA started rising, 3) patients with a slow PSA doubling time, and 4) patients with at least a 5 to 10 year life expectancy. We don't want to treat patients who have had a lot of radiation side effects in the past. A highly experienced operating team is always preferable, and patients are strongly advised to seek second and third opinions when exploring salvage treatment options.

When Should Hormonal Therapy Be Initiated?

During recent years there has been a growing enthusiasm for the early initiation of hormonal therapy for patients with advanced disease who are not eligible for any form of salvage therapy. Early initiation means starting hormonal therapy, especially combination hormonal therapy, before any symptoms of metastatic disease appear. Advocates of this approach point to those studies that indicate some degree of local control achieved with hormonal agents, slowing progression of the disease. It might appear to be common sense that because hormonal therapy lowers PSA, shrinks tumors and slows progression of the cancer, that it would also prolong life. But this may not be the case. Although the benefits of hormonal therapy for treating prostate cancer have been established, there is considerable controversy about how effective hormonal therapy may be at increasing survival.

Researchers remain divided on the optimal time to begin therapy, though recent studies favor early versus late initiation of hormonal therapy. The argument against early use of hormones rests on the fact that those who opt for early initiation will not be able to use hormonal therapy later when symptoms appear. By that time, the tumor may have become androgen-independent and refractory. After the beneficial effects of hormonal therapy have run their course, a patient's cancer may begin to grow again and eventually progress to what it would have been had hormonal therapy never been given. With this in mind, some doctors encourage men with advanced disease to embark on a course of active surveillance, arguing that these patients should avoid side effects as long as possible since the treatment has not been shown to substantially prolong life. This conservative strategy calls for the use of hormone therapy only if and when symptoms appear.

Other researchers argue that men with metastatic disease yet smaller tumors and low Gleason scores (less aggressive cancer) might even be cured if treatment is started sooner because these patients have less cancer to begin with and slower growing cancer. As a tumor grows and becomes bulky, genetic changes may take place within the cancer cells that lead to androgen-independence; therefore, early treatment might offer some advantage for these patients by attacking the cancer before it becomes refractory. This point of view is supported by a Mayo Clinic non-randomized study which indicated that patients with positive lymph nodes and low Gleason scores lived longer if they were treated hormonally before symptoms appeared.

Early initiation of hormonal therapy may indeed halt disease progression temporarily while these patients evaluate other primary treatment options. But a number of studies have demonstrated that early hormonal intervention prior to radical surgery does not reduce the risk of biochemical failure. However, the early use of hormones appears to be more advantageous before undertaking radiation as a primary therapy. Our own patients who received hormones had very aggressive tumors, and yet they fared similarly to those low risk patients who did not receive hormones. As the high risk group would have been expected to fare much worse, this would therefore support the use of hormones in this group. In addition, numerous multi-institutional studies both in the U.S. and abroad have demonstrated a benefit with the utilization of hormonal therapy prior to, during and after radiation (see the RTOG clinical trials cited below).

It is clear that more men regardless of the stage of their cancer are choosing to initiate hormonal therapy early because of a perceived possibility of cure, or long-term remission. This option may seem appealing given the steady progress in the field and the likely development of new and more effective chemical agents in the near future. However, before making this choice, patients should fully investigate the potential side effects and changes in quality of life that can be anticipated with hormonal manipulation. Men who opt for early combination hormonal therapy should also keep in mind that the hormones are likely to stop working eventually. Regardless of the stage of cancer, patients should also consider lifestyle changes, including diet and nutrition, and utilizing agents like Celebrex® and Zyflamend®.

Hormonal therapy continues to be controversial because there are still so many unanswered questions in this area, and because doctors disagree about what the answers will turn out to be. The nature of this controversy makes it all the more important for patients to question their doctors carefully before embarking on treatment. Be sure your doctor has considerable experience with hormonal therapy, and find out what that experience has been with other patients of similar age and stage of cancer as your own.

You should carefully discuss the pros and cons of each drug with your doctors and if you remain in doubt, by all means, obtain a second opinion. While the lack of definitive knowledge about hormonal therapy may be unsettling, each patient can still make an educated decision based on the possible benefits and risks associated with this form of treatment.

What Options Are Available Once Hormonal Therapy Stops Working?

All combinations of hormonal therapy should be completely exhausted before further therapeutic options are considered. For example, if the antiandrogen Casodex® ceases to be effective as indicated by a rising PSA, consideration might be given to changing to another antiandrogen such as Nilandron® or Androcur®. There are many hormonal options currently available and new drugs are constantly being developed for FDA-approval and clinical application.

For prostate cancer that becomes resistant to all combinations of hormonal therapy, chemotherapy agents such as Taxotere® (docetaxel) were long regarded by oncologists as the standard of care, though that assessment has changed dramatically during recent years. Doctors often administer chemo in 2 to 3 week cycles, with each period of treatment followed by a short break for patients to recover from the adverse side effects of those drugs.

Many patients resist undergoing chemotherapy because they see it as a short-term endgame, with limited survival benefits measured in months and severe side effects. The side effects of Taxotere® include hematological toxicities such as febrile neutropenia (low white blood cell count leading to infection and fever), which can be extremely debilitating, impacting about 10% of patients. As many as 60% or more of patients on Taxotere® develop peripheral neuropathy (short- or long-term peripheral nerve disease). Other potential side effects include fatigue, nausea, vomiting, diarrhea, hair loss, anemia, loss of appetite, mouth sores, bleeding, reduced heart function, and fluid retention. Some of these complications can be ameliorated with medications.

Another chemotherapy agent, Jevtana® (cabazitaxel), has been prescribed in recent years for hormone-resistant prostate cancer. This chemo agent may be prescribed when Taxotere® stops working or cannot be tolerated. Jevtana® has somewhat less overall toxicity than Taxotere®, although Jevtana® similarly impacts quality of life for many patients. Fewer patients who are prescribed Jevtana® suffer from neuropathy (less than 10%), fatigue and hair loss than those on Taxotere®; but a much higher percentage of patients experience neutropenia with Jevtana® (more than 90%).

One large study reported percentages of patients who experienced hematological and gastrointestinal toxicities with Jevtana® as follows: neutropenia (94%), anemia (97%), leukopenia (96%), thrombocytopenia (47%), diarrhea (47%), nausea (34%), and vomiting (22%). (Tsao CK, et al, The role of cabazitaxel in the treatment of metastatic castration-resistant prostate cancer; Ther Adv Urol. 2014 Jun;6 (3):97-104).

A number of newly developed therapies such as immunotherapy and therapeutic vaccines are currently being offered clinically as alternatives to chemotherapy, often with significant survival benefits and fewer and less severe side effects. At our center, when treating androgen-independent, advanced prostate cancer, we are increasingly utilizing genetic/genomic testing in order to create a "designer cocktail," which often includes an immunotherapy agent that may be given in conjunction with high-tech and infusional irradiation, with or without DART (Dynamic Adaptive Radiotherapy). Genetic markers help us determine which patients are likely to benefit from particular therapeutic agents. Genetic testing is becoming increasingly important, as is molecular profiling, to select the right drugs for the specific tumor.

A recent survey from the Memorial Sloan-Kettering Cancer Center suggests that immunotherapy agents for prostate cancer show enhanced benefits when utilized in combination with various biologic agents, vaccines, chemotherapies, and radiation (Slovin SF, Immunotherapy in metastatic prostate cancer, In J Urol. 2016 Oct-Dec; 32(4): 27-276).

When patients stop responding to hormonal therapy, we usually consider one of two FDA-approved drugs, Xtandi® (enzalutamide) and Zytiga® (abiraterone). These are androgen-blocking agents, and they have been shown to prolong survival, irrespective of age. Both of these drugs act to inhibit the production of testosterone and dihydrotestosterone in the prostate gland and elsewhere in the body, thereby lowering PSA and slowing the growth of prostate cancer. As a second-line therapy after ADT stops working, we often combine Xtandi® and prednisone. Prior to prescribing androgen-blocking agents such as Xtandi® and Zytiga®, we employ multiple lab tests for genomic makeup that allow us to determine which of these drugs may be appropriate for each patient.

At our center, we employ multiple laboratory tests for genomic and genetic makeup that allow us to determine which specific medications and treatments may be most appropriate for each patient. We utilize both the Invitae Genetic Test and the Myriad myRisk® Hereditary Cancer testing. The Myriad test is a 35-gene panel that identifies elevated risk for eight hereditary cancers. There are a host of genetic pathways and mutations that a patient may have (including BRACA 2, BRCA1, HOXB13, ATM, CHEK2, and CDK1), and they can tell us whether or not a patient is likely to respond well to a particular agent. For example, we know that a patient with positive BRCA1 and especially positive BRCA2 gene mutations will most likely have a shorter effective run with the androgen-blocking drugs Xtandi® and Zytiga®.

Another lab test analyzing serum is called a "droplet digital PCR assay," and it can also help us determine which patients will best respond to those chemical agents, Xtandi® and Zytiga®. It should be noted that genetic markers are also important in light of the patient's family history. We want to know what the family history is with regard to other cancers. We can see that a patient's daughters may be prone to breast cancer or ovarian cancer; and now we are seeing colon and pancreatic cancers enter the picture in the spectrum related to prostate cancer. These cancers are essentially on the same page in our genetic makeup. Melanoma is also genetically related to prostate cancer, and all of these cancers may occur at increased frequency in the patient tested.

While genetic testing is important for the patient's siblings and children, (and also for the patient on occasion), there is even greater importance in sampling the actual cancerous tissue removed from the patient in order to identify somatic mutations. This is known as comprehensive genomic profiling (CGP). This test can help identify exactly which particular treatment may benefit the patient. AR-7 mutations suggest resistance to Xtandi®/Zytiga® while HRR gene mutations predict response to Lynparza® (olaparib). Checkpoint inhibitors (e.g. PD-1) suggest sensitivity to pembrolizumab.

We have been using FoundationOne®CDx as the best genomic test currently available for identifying somatic mutations. This test searches 324 genes for cancer-relevant mutations in the DNA.

Both Xtandi® and Zytiga® have a side effect profile similar to that of hormonal therapy. In conjunction with these agents, we also use metaformin, which has an anti-cancer mechanism and has been shown to enhance the efficacy of Xtandi® and Zytiga®. Metaformin works in the pancreatic insulin pathway.

With patients for whom Xtandi® and Zytiga® are not effective or are unlikely to be effective as indicated by positive genetic markers (BRCA1 and BRCA2), we may prescribe Lynparza®, which is known as a PARP inhibitor (poly ADP-ribose polymerase). Many patients fare quite well with Lynparza®. Another immunotherapy agent, Keytruda® (pembrolizumab) is known as a PD1 inhibitor. We are finding that patients who are not responding well to Lynparza may benefit from Keytruda.

We have a growing arsenal of medications at our disposal for patients with advanced or recurrent disease. Both hormonal therapies and immunotherapies are associated with far less toxicity than chemotherapy, as they are "targeted therapies."

➤ For more information about the Myriad myRisk® Hereditary Cancer Test, visit online: https://myriad.com/products-services/hereditary-cancers/my-risk -hereditary-cancer/

➤ To learn more about Invitae Genetic Testing, visit online: https://www.invitae.com/en/detect-hereditary-prostate-cancer/

> The National Comprehensive Cancer Network (NCCN) offers patients recommendations on genetic testing and describes Medicare coverage here: https://myriad.com/products-services/hereditary-cancers/myrisk-hereditary-cancer/

> Additional information on the FDA approved FoundationOne ®CDx Test is available here: https://www.foundationmedicine.com/test/foundationone-cdx

The immunotherapy agent, Provenge® (sipuleucel-T) is a therapeutic vaccine that received FDA approval in 2010 for treating prostate cancer patients. While the reported overall survival improvement with this drug was only four months for patients with advanced disease, this positive development gave hope to many patients who had few options and were facing grim prospects at that time. We have come a long way since then. Research developing Provenge® soon led to a number of similar prostate cancer immunotherapeutic drugs that have also won FDA approval. Other novel therapeutic agents are now regularly being prescribed for hormone-refractory prostate cancer.

On July 30, 2019, another newly developed androgen-blocking agent, Nubeqa® (darolutamide), was approved by the FDA for the treatment of patients with castration-resistant prostate cancer that has not metastasized (nmCRPC). Most patients with castration-resistant prostate cancer have metastatic disease (mCRPC), so this agent has limited clinical application. On September 17, 2019, the FDA approved another androgen-blocking agent, Erleada® (apalutamide), for patients with metastatic castration-sensitive prostate cancer (mCSPC), a year after having been approved for treating non-metastatic, castration-resistant prostate cancer (nmCRPC).

As with enzalutamide and abiraterone, some studies have shown that apalutamide combined with ADT for newly diagnosed, advanced cancer patients achieves greater overall survival than ADT alone with patients starting hormonal therapy for the first time (Armstrong AJ, et al, ARCHES: A Randomized, Phase III Study of Androgen Deprivation Therapy With Enzalutamide or Placebo in Men With Metastatic Hormone-Sensitive Prostate Cancer, J Clin Oncol, 2019 Jul 22:JCO1900799; also see: Hoyle AP, et al, Abiraterone in "High-" and "Low-risk" Metastatic Hormone-sensitive Prostate Cancer, Eur Urol, 2019 Aug 22; S0302-2838(19)30620-7).

An FDA-approved infusional irradiation agent, Xofigo® (Radium-223) is an alpha particle radioisotope, which can be delivered to patients in a one-minute infusion and attacks prostate cancer that has spread to the bones. Not only does Xofigo® relieve bone pain, but it also improves overall survival (Parker C, et al, Efficacy and Safety of Radium-223 Dichloride in Symptomatic Castration-resistant Prostate

Cancer Patients With or Without Baseline Opioid Use From the Phase 3 ALSYMPCA Trial; Eur Urol, 2016 Nov; 70(5): 875-883).

Xofigo® is now being combined with Zytiga®, Xtandi® and Provenge®, and the combination appears to be synergistic. For patients with multiple bone metastases, we are having success with a 3X protocol combining Xgeva®, Xtandi®, and Xofigo®. For patients with visceral metastases (e.g. liver and/or lung) we may intervene with Zytiga® and prednisone. If metastases are confined to lymph nodes only, we stay with only intensive combination ADT, which usually brings PSA down to nadir value.

A large multi-institutional Phase III clinical trial reported that Zytiga® plus prednisone combined with ADT showed significantly improved survival versus ADT alone for patients with advanced disease: "Adding abiraterone acetate (Zytiga) plus prednisone to standard hormonal therapy for men newly diagnosed with high-risk, metastatic prostate cancer lowers the chance of death by 38%" (2017 American Society of Clinical Oncology (ASCO) Annual Meeting. press release, June 3, 2017; also see: Fizazi K, et al, Abiraterone acetate plus prednisone in patients with newly diagnosed high-risk metastatic castration-sensitive prostate cancer (LATITUDE): final overall survival analysis of a randomized, double-blind, phase 3 trial, Lancet Oncol, 2019 May;20(5):686-700. doi: 10.1016/S1470-2045(19)30082-8).

Both Xofigo® and Provenge® are expensive, as are Zytiga® and Xtandi®. Xofigo® costs more than $60,000 for six injections; and Provenge® costs more than $90,000 for three infusions. Zytiga® now retails for more than $9,000 per month; and the cost for Xtandi® is more than $12,000 for a 1-month supply of 120 capsules (40 mg). On our staff we have oncology nurses who try to work with insurance companies to make these agents more affordable for patients.

Whereas Xofigo® only treats bone, another injectable radioisotope, Actinium-225, attaches to prostate-specific membrane antigen (PSMA). PSMA is found on the surface of most metastatic prostate cancer cells. Therefore Actinium-225 treats not only bone, but also can target metastases in any tissue or fluid, even undetectable systemic micro-metastases. Since it is an alpha emitter (very short range), it is less toxic to bone marrow and other nearby tissues. Actinium-225 is currently in the pipeline and we hope it will be released soon (Kratochwil C, et al, 225Ac-PSMA-617 for PSMA targeting alpha-radiation therapy of patients with metastatic castration-resistant prostate cancer, J Nucl Med July 7, 2016). A similar agent, Lutetium-177 PSMA, has been FDA-approved but so far has only limited availability.

Xgeva® (denosumab) is a subcutaneous injection given monthly to treat bone metastases and to deter further bone metastases by blocking the glycoprotein known as RANKL (receptor activator nuclear factor ligand), which plays an important role in prostate cancer proliferation in bone. This agent is used in patients having documented spread to one or more bone sites. In this setting, patients receive 12 consecutive months of Xgeva® and then enter a 3-month holiday. Side effects with Xgeva® may include fatigue, weakness, headache, back and joint pain, diarrhea and nausea.

We are also currently using Xgeva® in patients without skeletal metastases in lower doses given once every 6 months to help strengthen the bones in prostate cancer patients who are on ADT, with the added potential benefit of deterring metastatic bone spread. Meanwhile we are awaiting the outcome of trials delivering Xgeva® monthly in patients having organ confined, high-risk non-metastatic prostate cancer (Smith MR, et al, Denosumab and bone-metastasis-free survival in men with castration-resistant prostate cancer, Lancet. 2012 Jan 7:379(9810): 39-460); also see: Miller K, et al, Harnessing the potential of therapeutic agents to safeguard bone health in prostate cancer; Prostate Cancer Prostatic Dis, 2018; 21(4): 461–472).

There is also a great deal of interest in combining immunotherapies with other therapeutic agents and especially radiation. Combining radiation with immunogenic drugs has great promise since the effects of the body's immune response to cancer is enhanced (Golden EB, et al Semin Radiat Oncol. 2015:25 (1) 7-11). These immunogenic synergistic effects of radiation and immunogenic drugs (especially those known as "checkpoint inhibitors" like PD1 and PARP inhibitors, and even Zytiga® and Xtandi®) are thought to result from 'autovaccination' by antigens released from dying cancer cells and fragmented, damaged DNA. Checkpoint inhibitors are immunotherapy agents that block certain proteins that stop the immune system from attacking the cancer cells.

Mechanistically, radiation (all types, including Xofigo.) has been shown to augment the afferent, as well as the efferent arms of cancer immunity. The induction of a positive T-cell immune response against cancer has been observed in numerous studies (Kapoor A, et al, Contemporary agents in the management of metastatic castration-resistant prostate cancer, Can Urol Assoc J. 2016 Nov-Dec;10(11-12):E414-E423).

There are novel immunotherapy agents that ramp up both T-cells and B-cells to attack prostate cancer cells. These are checkpoint inhibitors that encompass a class of drugs including anti-PD-1/PDL-1 inhibitors such as Opdivo® (nivolumab,) as well as anti-CTLA-4 inhibitors such as Yervoy® (ipilimumab). These immunotherapeutic checkpoint inhibitors are currently being used in other cancers and have been FDA-approved for melanoma, lung and kidney cancers. We are hopeful that checkpoint inhibitors and other novel therapies will be "fast tracked" by the FDA, similar to the experience with Zytiga® and Xtandi®.

The biomarker Androgen Receptor Splice Varient-7 (AR-V7) expression in tissue, and more recently in blood, could predict resistance to Zytiga® and Xtandi®, and it could help personalize checkpoint inhibitors. AR-V7 may also possibly allow for chemotherapy to be more specifically designed for the tumor. We eagerly await AR-V7 winning FDA approval (Antonarakis ES, et al, Clinical Significance of Androgen Receptor Splice Variant-7 mRNA Detection in Circulating Tumor Cells of Men with Metastatic Castration-Resistant Prostate Cancer Treated with First- and Second-Line Abiraterone and Enzalutamide, J Clin Oncol. 2017 Apr 6; also see: Scher HI, et al, Association of AR-V7 on Circulating Tumor Cells as a Treatment-Specific Biomarker with Outcomes and Survival in Castration-Resistant Prostate Cancer, JAMA Oncol. 2016 Nov 1;2(11):1441-1449).

Finally, it should also be noted that while ADT and other therapeutic agents are important in treating metastatic disease, we have long been proponents of treating the primary tumor with external radiation, preferably DART. A number of studies have demonstrated that treating the primary tumor site with radiotherapy significantly improves overall survival for patients with metastatic prostate cancer. A recent multi-institutional position paper suggested this should be the standard of care for treating metastatic disease (Choudhury A, et al, STAMPEDE: Is Radiation Therapy to the Primary a New Standard of Care in Men with Metastatic Prostate Cancer? Int J Radiat Oncol Biol Phys, 2019 May 1;104(1):33-35).

What Have We Learned?

✔ PSA Matters—Don't let it get too high

✔ Dose Matters—Higher doses are more effective

✔ Adjuvant vs Salvage Radiation Matters

✔ Time to PSA Relapse Matters

✔ Grade Matters

✔ Meticulous re-staging work-up is essential

✔ Lower pre-salvage PSA is associated with favorable outcome

✔ Use of neo-adjuvant hormonal therapy enables us to achieve maximal downsizing and radio-sensitization, with use of adjunctive and adjuvant hormones

✔ We attenuate the implant dose, for example:
PD-103 10,000 to 11,000 cGy (vs. 12,500 cGy)

✔ I-125 11,000 to 12,000 cGy (vs. 14,400 cGy)

Other

✔ Seminal Vesicle involvement Matters

✔ Using a higher does with more sophisticated radiation modalities (beyond IMRT) while lowering toxicity

✔ Exploit the synergistic effects of radiation combined with hormones

✔ The sophistication of the radiation technique matters (beyond IMRT) with increasing dose levels, because dose is crucially important

FREQUENTLY
ASKED QUESTIONS

1. At what point can I stop worrying and consider myself cured?

If you have had a radical prostatectomy (open or robotic or laparoscopic surgery) and if you have been disease-free for more than 10 years, then you can be somewhat confident that your cancer will not return, though as discussed there are still treatment failures with surgery in the long term. Surgical patients in the intermediate and high risk before treatment categories still have a risk of a recurrence at 10 or more years after treatment. In general, this perspective on disease-free survival also applies to patients who have had conventional external radiation therapy or 3D-Conformal Radiation Therapy, as well as to patients who have undergone therapies that are less widely used, such as HDR brachytherapy, Proton Beam Therapy, and cryosurgery.

Patients who have undergone IMRT alone are probably wise to be cautiously optimistic over a similar time span. While we expect results with DART to be superior to those obtained by other forms of external radiation, we do not yet have 10-year studies because the technology utilized with this procedure is still relatively new. Based on our research and the published results of other brachytherapy teams, seed implant patients who have not experienced biochemical failure at six years or more can be reasonably confident that the cancer will not recur, though there are some long term failures. With our brachytherapy patients, including those who received supplemental external radiation (either 3D-CRT or DART), most of those who failed did so within 3 years after treatment. There is probably no absolute time limit to rule out recurrence with any treatment, but we are seeing very few failures beyond 6 years.

2. How often do I need to go for a checkup after my initial treatment to see if there has been a recurrence?

The follow-up monitoring schedule varies somewhat depending on the type of treatment you received and according to the specifics of your individual case. Most patients will be checked every 3 to 6 months for the first year after treatment, and annually or biannually after that.

3. What are the signs of recurrence?

A relapse is generally detected by monitoring with PSA and DRE, and at our institution, with Color-Flow Power Doppler Ultrasound and other tests such as Dynamic Contrast Enhanced MRI along with various Fusion studies. After radiation and other non-surgical therapies, a rising PSA over time may signal a recurrence, or PSA that fails to reach a predetermined nadir value. After surgery, any PSA reading above zero may be a sign of recurrence, though many surgeons use PSA of 0.2 as the nadir value.

4. Can I transmit cancer cells to my partner through sexual activity?

No, prostate cancer is not in any way contagious.

5. Will an increase or decrease in sexual activity increase or decrease the risk of recurrence?

No, sexual activity does not increase or decrease the risk of recurrent cancer.

6. Can prostate cancer cause another type of cancer to form in another part of the body (ie. lungs, colon, blood)?

Prostate cancer cannot cause any other form of cancer. When prostate cancer metastasizes to the bones or some other part of the body, it is still prostate cancer, due to the fact that it originated in the prostate gland and retains the particular characteristics of this type of cancer. It cannot generate another kind of cancer in another part of the body (such as lung cancer or leukemia).

7. Should my wife be concerned that I may transmit cancer cells to her that might cause her to have ovarian, breast or some other type of cancer?

No, there is no cause for concern in that regard.

8. If my prostate becomes enlarged following my initial treatment, does that mean the cancer has recurred?

Not necessarily, but your doctor may recommend further tests beyond PSA, such Color-Flow Power Doppler Ultrasound or a prostate biopsy, to determine the cause of the enlargement.

9. If I have an increase in urination, or difficulty in urination, does that mean the cancer has recurred?

Short term urinary problems often occur following surgery or radiation, and in that circumstance, they do not indicate a recurrence. There are medications that are quite effective in treating these temporary urinary problems. You should make your doctor aware of any discomfort or burning or increased frequency of urination. If symptoms occur after the immediate post-treatment recovery period, further tests may be necessary to check for residual or recurrent disease. It is not uncommon to have temporary episodes (prostatitis) years after treatment.

10. Are there any drugs that are taken for other medical reasons (i.e. heart or blood pressure mediations) that increase the likelihood of recurrence?

Medications for other conditions should have no effect on the likelihood of recurrence; however, you should always inform your doctor of all other medications you are taking. Testosterone supplements should be avoided.

11. What can I do to reduce my chances of recurrence?

Devote yourself to maintaining a healthy, active lifestyle. Eat a balanced diet, one that is high in fiber and low in saturated fats. The benefits of some of the more radical dietary supplements are doubtful, but it is clear that the healthier you are in mind and body, the better you will be at fighting this disease through the recovery process. There are a number of specific antioxidants, phytochemicals and vitamins that may be beneficial for men with prostate cancer, but the practice of "mega-dosing" (taking more than RDA-recommended doses) should be avoided, or undertaken only under a doctor's supervision. *It should also be noted that patients undergoing radiation therapy should avoid excessive antioxidants while being treated, as these may have an opposing action to radiation.*

Suggested dietary guidelines and recipes for cancer patients are available from the National Cancer Institute (call the Cancer Information Service: 1-800-4-CANCER or visit the NCI Web site: http://cis.nci.nih.gov/). At our center, we provide patients with our own recommended nutrition/vitamin/supplement list that can be individualized for each patient.

Prostate enlargement due to benign prostatic hypertrophy (BPH) can cause the PSA to rise, as can prostatic infections (prostatitis). Both of these conditions can be effectively treated and do not indicate cancer. Temporary changes in the PSA can also be caused by the following:

➤ Trauma such as biopsy or overly vigorous digital rectal examination (DRE)

➤ Ejaculation (a 40 percent elevation, returning to normal within 48 hours)

➤ Strenuous exercise involving the buttocks or perineum (such as bicycle riding)

➤ Medical procedures such as balloon dilation of the prostate, transrectal ultrasound-guided biopsy, and transurethral resection of the prostate (TURP)

> Medications such as finasteride (Proscar®) used to treat BPH can decrease PSA levels by as much as 50 percent.

> Certain herbal mixtures marketed "for prostate health" may also affect PSA levels.

13. What is a PSA bounce, and is it a sign of recurrence?

About 30% to 40% of patients undergoing seed implantation experience a temporary rise in PSA after an initial decline in their PSA level following treatment. This phenomenon is known as a PSA bounce or flare. It usually occurs approximately 18 to 24 months after treatment and is not caused by a recurrence of cancer, but rather by radiation-induced prostatitis (inflammation of the prostate) with subsequent systemic release of PSA. These patients are still considered disease-free. The rise in PSA may be 0.1 or higher and can sometimes last many months, but it is usually of short duration. Studies have shown that the PSA bounce is more common with younger patients, those who receive higher implant doses, and those with larger prostate glands.

14. How often and when should I have a biopsy?

A biopsy is usually called for whenever there is a question of residual or recurrent cancer. A suspicious DRE or a rising PSA after initial treatment may warrant a biopsy and further testing. At our institution, we utilize additional tests such as Color-Flow Power Doppler Ultrasound, Dynamic Contrast Enhanced MRI, and other advanced imaging tests prior to or in conjunction with a biopsy.

15. Besides the PSA and DRE, should I have a bone scan, CT scan or biopsy if there is no rise in my PSA and my DRE is normal?

A prostate biopsy, CT scan, MRT and bone scan (PET) are used to check for the spread of cancer after treatment usually when there is some definite question of local or distant failure. A CT scan may also be used after brachytherapy to check on the placement of the seeds. Periodic post-treatment monitoring usually consists of the PSA test and DRE. As mentioned, at our institution, we also utilize Color-Flow Power Doppler Ultrasound and helical CT scans for monitoring.

16. Why did radical prostatectomy work for my friend but not for me?

Each case of prostate cancer has to be evaluated according to the individual patient's work-up and diagnostic history. What works for one patient may not work for another, even though the two patients may be very similar as far as the stage and grade of cancer. In the case of surgery, results can vary widely depending on the skill and experience of the surgeon, and the quality of services available at the hospital or medical center where the operation was performed.

17. Why did radiation work for my friend but not for me?

The same individual considerations hold true for radiation therapy as for surgery. Each man is different, and the results of all curative treatments can vary with different patients. You really can't depend on a friend's good or bad experience with a particular treatment. The wiser course is to check carefully on the published results of the leading practitioners within each specialty and on the results of your own physician with any particular treatment. Success rates should be weighed carefully against the risk of side effects with each type of therapy.

18. Would hormonal therapy reduce my risk of having a recurrence?

Hormonal therapy can interrupt the progression of the disease and to some extent delay a recurrence of prostate cancer. In the most cases, hormonal therapy would not be considered unless there is evidence of recurrence. It can be used in conjunction with a curative therapy such as radiation, if indicated, or it can be used as a palliative treatment for advanced disease. The effectiveness varies considerably from man to man as some cancers are resistant to hormonal therapy. For more information on this subject, readers are referred to the Prostate Cancer Essentials booklet, Hormonal Therapy for Prostate Cancer: The Benefits and Risks.

Questions To Ask Your Doctor

1. What makes you think a recurrence has occurred?

2. Is this a local or distant recurrence?

3. What tests will you do to confirm a recurrence?

4. What are my treatment options at this point?

5. What are the risks associated with each option?

6. How long can I take to come to a decision?

7. Given my age and the stage of the cancer, do I really need further treatment?

8. Will my lifestyle be affected?

9. When will I know if I'm cured?

10. Will you make my medical reports and test results available to me if I decide to seek a second opinion?

DECIDING WHAT IS BEST FOR YOU

Consult with your physician, and by all means, obtain second and third opinions whenever possible, preferably from physicians with different specialties. If you have already been to a urologist, it is worthwhile to visit a radiation oncologist or medical oncologist (those with experience with hormones and chemotherapy).

Join a support group such as US TOO!, or PAACT. If you belong to any of the computer on-line services, check out the medical and health bulletin boards and mailing lists for the latest information and announcements for prostate cancer patients. Keep your personal plan of action updated.

What to Remember

> Obtain all of the advice and counsel that you can, but keep in mind that the decisions are ultimately yours to make.

> Be positive—if you have been properly staged and treated, the odds are in your favor on not having a recurrence.

> If you should have a rising PSA over time after initial treatment, don't panic. Get further tests, and if appropriate, get a biopsy, preferably guided by Color-Flow Power Doppler Ultrasound.

> The secret to success with prostate cancer is catching the disease early, and that is also true for recurrence.

> If testing confirms cancer, learn all you can about your options. Get second and third opinions. Become informed and empowered. Become involved with solving your problem. It's your life and body. Go for it!

➤ Life is full of problems and challenges. Solve this problem like any other big problem:

1 Identify the problem.

2 Get all the facts to confirm that you have a problem.

3 Learn what options are available to you and weigh them carefully.

4 Choose a qualified doctor who is experienced and with whom you are comfortable.

5 Initiate and follow through with the solution.

➤ Don't be afraid to ask for help from your spouse or partner, from your family and your friends. It is more important than ever for you to turn to loved ones to get the emotional and spiritual support you need. This disease can be a difficult struggle for you, but you are not alone, and your mental attitude, prayers and fighting spirit really can make all the difference.

To be a cancer survivor, you must first be a cancer fighter!

GLOSSARY OF MEDICAL TERMS

3D-CRT (3-Dimensional Conformal Radiation Therapy): See Conformal Radiotherapy.

5-alpha reductase (5-AR): an enzyme that converts testosterone to dihydrotestosterone (DHT).

Adenocarcinoma: A cancer originating in glandular tissue. Prostate cancer is classified as adenocarcinoma of the prostate.

Adjuvant: An additional treatment used to increase the effectiveness of the primary therapy. Radiation therapy and hormonal therapy are often used as adjuvant treatments following a radical prostatectomy. Compare Neoadjuvant.

Agonist: A chemical substance that combines with a receptor on a cell and initiates an activity or reaction. See LHRH analogs.

Algorithm: A step-by-step procedure for solving a problem or accomplishing some end, especially by a computer.

Analog: A man-made chemical compound that is structurally similar to one produced naturally by the body. See LHRH analogs.

Anastomotic stricture: narrowing, usually by scarring, of an anastomotic suture line.

Androgen: A hormone that produces male characteristics. See testosterone.

Androgen ablation therapy: A therapy designed to inhibit the body's production of testosterones.

Androgen-dependent cells: Prostate cancer cells which are nourished by male hormones and therefore are capable of being destroyed by hormone deprivation (also known as androgen-sensitive cells).

Androgen-independent cells: Prostate cancer cells which are not dependent on male hormones and therefore do not respond to hormonal therapy (also known as androgen-insensitive cells).

Anesthetic: A drug that produces general or local loss of physical sensations, particularly pain. A "spinal" is the injection of a local anesthetic into the area surrounding the spinal cord.

Aneuploid: Having an abnormal number of chromosomes, as revealed by ploidy analysis. Aneuploid prostate cancer cells tend not to respond well to androgen deprivation therapy (ADT).

Angiogenesis: The body's formation of new blood vessels. Some anti-cancer drugs work by blocking angiogenesis, thus preventing blood from reaching and nourishing a tumor.

Antagonist: A chemical substance in the body that acts to reduce the physiological activity of another chemical substance.

Antiandrogens: Drugs such as Casodex that block the activity of androgens produced by the adrenal glands at the cellular receptor sites. Androgens can block or neutralize the effects of testosterone and DHT on prostate cancer cells.

Antibody: A protein produced by the body that counteracts the toxic effects of a foreign substance, organism, or disease within the body.

Antigen: A foreign substance such as a virus or bacterium that causes an immune response or the formation of an antibody.

Antineoplastic: Inhibits growth and proliferation of cancer cells.

Antioxidants: Any substances which delay the process of oxidation in the body.

Apoptosis: The normal molecular mechanism which governs the life span of cells so that they die in a very organized way. Cancerous cells are resistant to normal apoptosis.

Benign: A non-cancerous condition. See also Benign Prostatic Hypertrophy.

Benign Prostatic Hypertrophy (BPH): Also called Benign Prostatic Hyperplasia, BPH is a non-cancerous condition of the prostate that results in a growth of tumorous tissue and increase in the size of the prostate.

Biopsy: A procedure involving the removal of tissue from the body of the patient. Removed tissue is typically examined microscopically by a pathologist in order to make a precise diagnosis of the patient's condition.

Bone scan: An imaging technique used to detect bone metastases, which appear as "hot spots" on the film. It is far more sensitive than the conventional x-ray.

BPH: See Benign Prostatic Hypertrophy.

Brachytherapy: A form of radiation therapy in which radioactive seeds are implanted into the prostate to deliver radiation directly to the tumor. Also referred to as seed implantation, or seeding.

Cancer: A cellular malignancy typically forming tumors. Unlike benign tumors, these tend to invade surrounding tissues and spread to distant sites of the body.

Carcinoma: A malignant tumor made up chiefly of epithelial cells, or those cells that form the lining of an organ or cavity. See Adenocarcinoma.

Castrate Range: The level of the body's testosterone after orchiectomy (also referred to as castration). This is the range or level, which is used by physicians as a point of comparison for those drugs, which attempt to decrease the testosterone level.

CAT Scan (or CT Scan): See Computer Tomography.

cGy: Abbreviation for centigray; a unit of radiation equivalent to the older unit called a "rad."

Chemotherapy: The treatment of cancer using chemicals that deter the growth of cancer cells.

Collimator: A device that organizes radiation such that only parallel rays or beams emanate.

Combination Hormonal Therapy (CHT): Also referred to as Combined Hormonal Blockade (CHB), or Combined Androgen Deprivation Therapy (ADT). The preferred term is ADT, often designated with a number referring to the number of agents used (i.e., monotherapy ADT, ADT2, ADT3). This combined therapy can utilize a number of mechanisms, including surgical or medical ADT, antiandrogens, 5-alpha reductase inhibitors, estrogenic compounds, agents that block adrenal androgen production, and agents that decrease the receptivity of the androgen receptor.

Combination Therapy: Refers generally to any combination of treatment modalities used to treat prostate cancer.

Computer Tomography: Computer generated cross-sectional images of a portion of the body. Also called CT or CAT scan.

Conformal Radiotherapy: A radiation treatment conforming precisely to the size and shape of the prostate, with the use of computerized planning and state-of-the-art imaging techniques. 3-Dimensional Conformal Radiation Therapy (3D-CRT) utilizes this sophisticated approach to treatment planning, as does the even more advanced Intensity Modulated Radiation Therapy (IMRT).

Cryosurgery (also referred to as Cryotherapy or Cryoablation): The freezing of tissue with the use of liquid nitrogen or Argon gas probes. When used to treat prostate cancer, the cryoprobes are guided by transrectal ultrasound.

Cytokine: Any of a class of immuno-regulatory substances that are secreted by cells of the immune system.

DHT (dihydrotestosterone): The active form of the male hormone, testosterone, produced after testosterone is transformed by an enzyme known as 5-alpha reductase.

Diagnosis: Evaluation of a patient's symptoms and/or test results, with the intent of identifying and verifying the existence of any underlying disease or abnormal condition.

Digital Rectal Examination (DRE): A procedure in which the physician inserts a gloved, lubricated finger into the rectum to examine the prostate gland for signs of cancer.

DNA (Deoxyribonucleic Acid): A complex protein that is the carrier of genetic information that determines the physical development and growth of living organisms.

Doppler Ultrasound Technique: A machine that sends out ultrasonic waves that pick up the velocity of blood flow through the veins and are transmitted as sound to make an image.

Doubling Time: The time it takes for a tumor or cancerous focus to double in size.

Downsizing: The use of hormonal therapy or other forms of intervention to reduce tumor volume prior to primary, curative treatment.

Downstaging: The use of hormonal therapy or other forms of intervention to lower the clinical stage of prostate cancer prior to primary, curative treatment.

Ejaculatory Ducts: The tubular passages through which semen reaches the prostatic urethra during orgasm.

Ejaculation: The release of semen through the penis during orgasm.

Endorectal MRI: Magnetic resonance imaging of the prostate gland using a probe inserted into the rectum. Dynamic Contrast Enhanced MRI is the most effective form of magnetic resonance imaging.

Enzyme: A chemical substance produced by living cells that causes chemical reactions to take place while not being changed itself.

Erectile Dysfunction (also referred to as ED or impotence): The loss of ability to produce and/or sustain an erection sufficient for intercourse.

Estrogen: A female sex hormone that can be used as a form of therapy to inhibit the production of testosterone in patients diagnosed with prostate. cancer.

External Beam Radiation Therapy (EBRT): A form of radiation therapy that utilizes radiation delivered by an external source (machine) and directed at a target area to be radiated. In contrast to EBRT, brachytherapy utilizes radiation sources (seeds) that are internal, implanted in the target tissue. EBRT may use conventional photons, protons, neutrons or electrons.

Extraprostatic Extension: Used to describe prostate cancer that has spread outside the prostate gland.

False Negative: An erroneous negative test result. For example, an imaging test that fails to show the presence of a cancer tumor later found by biopsy to be present in the patient is said to have returned a false negative result.

False Positive: A positive test result that mistakenly identifies a state or condition that does not in fact exist.

Feraheme (Ferumoxytol): A ferromagnetic nanoparticle which is taken up by normal macrophages with the lymph nodes.

Fistula: With regard to prostate cancer, an abnormal passage due to injury or disease that connects an abscess or hollow organ to the surface of the body or to another hollow organ. If there is significant damage to the rectal wall proximate to the bladder, a fistula may occur between the bladder and rectum.

Flare Reaction: A testosterone surge caused by the initial use of an LHRH analog, causing a temporary increase of tumor growth and symptoms (known as clinical flare), or an increase in PSA (biochemical flare).

Foley Catheter: A catheter inserted in the penis and threaded through the urethra to the bladder where it is held in place with a tiny, inflated balloon. It removes urine from the bladder and can be used to irrigate the urethra and prevent blood clots.

Free PSA: PSA that is unattached to any major protein in the blood. Free PSA is associated with benign prostate growth. The percentage of free PSA is derived by dividing the free-PSA level by the total-PSA x 100. Studies have show that men with free PSA % > 25% were at low risk for prostate cancer, while men with PSA % < 10% were at high risk for having prostate cancer.

Frozen Section: A technique in which removed tissue is frozen, cut into thin slices, and stained for microscopic examination. A pathologist can rapidly complete a frozen section analysis, and for this reason, it is commonly used during surgery to quickly provide the surgeon with vital information.

Gland: An aggregation of cells (a structure or organ) that secretes a substance for use or discharge from the body.

Gland Volume: The size in cubic centimeters (cc) or grams of the prostate gland.

Gleason Score: A widely used method for classifying the cellular differentiation of cancerous tissue. The less the cancerous cells appear like normal cells, the more malignant the cancer. Two grades of 1-5, identifying the two most common degrees of differentiation present in the examined tissue sample, are added together to produce the Gleason score. High numbers indicate greater differentiation and more aggressive cancer. The grading system is named after its originator, Donald Gleason, M.D.

Globulin: Any of a number of simple proteins that occur widely in plant and animal tissues.

Gynecomastia: A side effect involving breast enlargement and tenderness, associated with various hormonal therapies that increase the level of estrogens in the body.

HDR brachytherapy: High Dose Rate brachytherapy involves the temporary insertion of radioactive iridium isotopes into the prostate gland using transrectal ultrasound guidance.

Hematuria: Blood in the urine.

Hereditary: Inherited genetically from parents and earlier generations.

Holistic Medicine: Medical care, which considers the patient as a whole, including his or her physical, mental, emotional, spiritual, social and economic needs.

Hormone: A substance produced by one tissue or gland and transported by the bloodstream to another to effect or regulate physiological activity such as metabolism and growth.

Hormonal therapy: Cancer treatment involving the blockage of hormone production by surgical or chemical means. Because prostate cancer is usually dependent on male hormones to grow, hormonal therapy can be an effective means of alleviating symptoms and retarding the development of the disease.

Hormone refractory prostate cancer: Prostate cancer that is androgen independent, and therefore, unresponsive to hormonal therapies.

Hot Flash: A side effect of some forms of hormonal therapy, experienced as a sudden rush of warmth to the face, neck, and upper body.

Imaging: Radiology techniques that are often computer-enhanced and allow the physician to visualize areas inside the body that would not normally be visible.

Impotence: See Erectile Dysfunction.

Incontinence: A loss of urinary control. There are various kinds and degrees of incontinence. Overflow incontinence is a condition in which the bladder retains urine after voiding. As a consequence, the bladder remains full most of the time, resulting in involuntary seepage of urine from the bladder. Stress incontinence is the involuntary discharge of urine when there is increased pressure upon the bladder, as in coughing or straining to lift heavy objects. Total incontinence is the failure of ability to voluntarily exercise control over the sphincters of the bladder neck and urethra, resulting in total loss of retentive ability.

Inflammation: Redness or swelling caused by injury or infection.

Informed Consent: Permission to proceed given by a patient after being fully informed of the purposes and potential consequences of a medical procedure.

Intensity Modulated Radiation Therapy (IMRT): The most recent state-of-the-art, computer-aided technique for delivering higher doses of radiation more accurately than either conventional External Beam Radiation or Conformal Radiation. The most advanced form of IMRT is Dynamic Adaptive Radiotherapy (DART).

Intermittent Androgen Deprivation (IAD): A temporary discontinuation of hormonal therapy that allows for a return to natural testosterone production in order to spare the patient from symptoms associated with androgen deprivation. Also referred to as Intermittent Hormonal Therapy (IHT).

Intravenous Pyelogram (IVP): A test that utilizes the injection of a special dye to check for injury or the spread of cancer to the kidneys and bladder.

Investigational: A drug or procedure allowed by the FDA for use in clinical trails, but not necessarily reimbursed.

Isodose Line: A line or two-dimensional shape that circumscribes an area receiving a radiation dose greater than or equal to a specified amount.

Laparoscopic Lymphadenectomy: The removal of pelvic lymph nodes with a laparoscope via four small incisions in the lower abdomen.

LH (Luteinizing Hormone): A chemical signal originating in the pituitary gland that causes the testes to make testosterone.

LHRH Analogs (or LHRH Agonists): Synthetic compounds that are chemically similar to Luteinizing Hormone Releasing Hormone (LHRH), used to suppress testicular production of testosterone. The most commonly prescribed LHRH analogs are Lupron® and Zoldex® Eligard® and Trelstar®. See also Luteinizing Hormone-Releasing Hormone (LHRH).

LHRH Antagonist: A chemical agent that blocks the LHRH receptor without the testosterone surge associated with

LHRH analogs. LHRH antagonists include Abarelix (Plenaxis®).

Linear Accelerator: A high energy x-ray machine generating radiation fields for external beam radiation therapy. These machines are typically mounted with a collimator (or multileaf collimator) in a gantry that rotates vertically around the patient being treated.

Localized Prostate Cancer: Cancer that is confined to the prostate gland, and therefore, considered curable.

Luteinizing Hormone-Releasing Hormone (LHRH): A chemical signal originating in the hypothalamus that causes the pituitary to make LH, which in turn stimulates the testicles to make testosterone.

Lymphadenectomy: The removal and examination of lymph nodes to precisely diagnose and stage cancer. See also Laparascopic Lymphadenectomy.

Lymph Node: A small, bean-shaped mass of tissue located throughout the body along the vessels of the lymphatic system. The lymph nodes filter out bacteria and other toxins, as well as cancer cells.

Magnetic Resonance Imaging (MRI): A painless, non-invasive technique using strong magnetic fields to produce detailed images of internal body structures. An MRI scan usually takes about 45 minutes per site.

Malignancy: A tumorous growth of cancer cells.

Malignant: Having the invasive and metastatic properties of cancer. Tending to become progressively worse and to result in death.

Margin: See Surgical Margin.

Metalloprotease Inhibitors: Drugs used to suppress the body's production of certain enzymes.

Metastasis: The spread of cancer, by way of the blood stream or lymphatic system, beyond the boundaries of the organ or structure where the cancer originated. Metastases is the plural. Metastatic refers to the characteristics associated with cancer that has spread or a secondary tumor.

Metastatic Work-Up: A group of tests, including bone scans, x-rays, and blood tests, to ascertain whether cancer has metastasized.

Monoclonal Antibody (mAb): An antibody that is directed against one specific protein (antigen).

Morbidity: Unhealthy consequences and complications resulting from treatment.

MRI: See Magnetic Resonance Imaging.

Nadir: The lowest point. Doctors sometimes use this as a verb to describe return of cancer or treatment failure. The PSA nadir refers to a minimum PSA value that should be maintained after treatment if the cancer has been successfully eradicated.

Necrosis: Death of cells or tissues caused by disease or injury.

Neoadjuvant: The use of a different type of therapy before primary, curative treatment. For example, neoadjuvant Androgen Deprivation Therapy is often used prior to radiation therapy or radical surgery, with the intent of improving the effectiveness of the primary treatment by reducing the size of the tumor and/ or prostate gland.

Nerve-sparing: A procedure used during radical prostatectomy in which the surgeon attempts to save the nerves (neurovascular bundles) that allow for normal sexual functions.

Neurovascular Bundles: Strands of interwoven nerves and veins that run down the side of the prostate. The bundles contain microscopic nerves that are essential for erection; they also contain arteries and veins. Cutting the nerves in the bundles during surgery, or otherwise harming them in another procedure, usually renders the patient impotent.

Nocturia: Getting up at night to urinate.

Non-invasive: Not involving any incision in the body.

Oncogenes: Genes associated with tumor growth.

Oncology: The branch of medical science dealing with tumors. A medical oncologist is a specialist in the study of cancerous tumors.

Organ-confined Disease (OCD): Prostate cancer that is confined to the prostate gland, as indicated clinically or pathologically.

Orchiectomy: A simple operation that involves surgical removal of the testicles, which produce most of the body's testosterone.

Osteoporosis: A decrease in bone mass and density causing fragility and porosity.

Overstaging: An assessment of an overly high clinical stage at initial diagnosis.

Palliative: Affording symptomatic pain relieve but not cure or remission.

Palpable: Capable of being felt when examined by touch or manipulation.

PAP: See Prostatic Acid Phosphatase.

Pathologist: A doctor who specializes in the examination of cells and tissues removed from the body.

PBRT: See Proton Beam Radiation Therapy.

Perineum: The area of the body between the anus and scrotum. A perineal procedure uses this area as the point of entry into the body.

Perineural Invasion: Describing cancer, which has spread from the prostate to the nerve bundles.

Periprostatic: Relating to the soft tissues immediately proximate to the prostate gland.

Photon: The quantum of electromagnetic energy, described as having zero mass and no electric charge. X-rays are high energy photons.

Placebo: A sugar pill often taken by participants in a medical study. Patients taking a placebo are compared to patients taking actual medications.

Ploidy Analysis: A pathological analysis to determine the number of sets of chromosomes in a cell.

Proctitis: Inflammation of the rectum.

Prognosis: A forecast of the course of a disease and future prospects of the patient.

Progression: A change in the status of the cancer indicating the condition has progressed and worsened.

Pro-oxidant: A term to describe substances that aid in oxidation.

ProstaScint® Scan: An imaging technique sometimes used determine whether or not cancer has spread to distant sites by using monoclonal antibodies.

Prostate Capsule: It was once thought that the prostate gland was surrounded by a clearly identifiable capsule, but pathological studies have shown there is no capsule as such. The gland exists within a fat plane.

Prostatectomy: The surgical removal of part or all of the prostate gland.

Prostate Specific Antigen (PSA): A blood test that measures a substance manufactured solely by prostate gland cells. An elevated reading indicates an abnormal condition of the prostate gland, either benign or malignant. It is presently the most sensitive tumor marker for the identification and monitoring of prostate cancer.

Prostatic Acid Phosphatase (PAP): An enzyme produced by the prostate that is elevated (3.0 or higher) in many patients when prostate cancer has spread beyond the prostate.

Prostatitis: An infection or inflammation of the prostate gland that is treatable with medications.

Proton Beam Radiation Therapy (PBRT): A form of radiation therapy that utilizes protons as the source of energy (as opposed to X-rays or neutrons).

PSA: See Prostate Specific Antigen.

PSA Bounce (or PSA Bump): A rise in PSA level after first having a reduction in PSA after radiation therapy.

PSA Nadir: The lowest PSA value after a particular treatment.

PSA Velocity (PSAV): The rate of increase of the PSA level, expressed as nanograms per milliliter per year.

Radiation Therapy (RT): The use of high energy rays to kill cancer cells and malignant tissue.

Radiation Urethritis: Inflammation of the urethra caused by radiation therapy.

Radical Prostatectomy: An operation to remove the entire prostate gland and seminal vesicles.

Radiosensitivity: The degree to which a type of cancer responds to radiation therapy.

RBA or Relative Biological Effectiveness: A scale used to compare the intensity of radiation associated with various atomic particles.

Receptor: A cellular docking site that interacts with a specific protein or enzyme (called a ligand). The interaction typically leads to the synthesis of other substances such as proteins, hormones or enzymes.

Recurrence: Return of the cancer following remission or treatment intended as curative. Local recurrence indicates a return of the cancer at the site of origin. Distant recurrence indicates the appearance of one or more metastases of the disease.

Refractory: A term indicating that the cancer no longer responds to the current therapy.

Remission: Complete or partial disappearance of the signs and symptoms of the disease. The period during which a disease remains under control, without progressing. Even complete remission does not necessarily indicate cure.

Resection: The surgical removal of a part of an organ or structure.

Risk: The probability that a particular event will or will not happen.

RP: See Radical Prostatectomy.

RT: See Radiation Therapy.

Rx: The standard abbreviation for prescription.

Salvage Treatment: A medical term for "Plan B." It means a patient must undergo another form of treatment because the first therapy was not successful. Salvage therapy may incur a higher rate of side effects.

Saw Palmetto: A nutrient extracted from the saw palmetto shrub, which is considered by some to aid the body's immune system.

Seed Implantation (SI): A minimally invasive procedure by which radioactive seeds are implanted into the prostate gland to destroy cancer. Also referred to as seeding and brachytherapy.

Selenium: A non-metallic element thought to be beneficial as a nutrient; it is often included in multivitamin supplements.

Seminal Vesicles: Glands that, like the prostate, support male reproduction. Fluid secreted by these glands regulates the consistency of semen.

Side Effect: A reaction to a treatment or medication, usually referring to an undesirable effect.

Sphincter: A circular muscle which contracts to close an orifice. The urethral sphincter squeezes the urethra shut, providing urinary control.

Staging: The testing process by which the extent and severity of a known cancer is evaluated according to an established system of classification. It is used to help determine appropriate therapy. See TNM Staging and Whitmore-Jewett Staging.

Surgical Margin: The outer edge of the tissue removed during a radical prostatectomy. The surgical margin may be "negative," indicating that no cancer is present and a better prognosis, or "positive," indicating that not all of the cancer has been removed.

Systemic: Throughout the body and affecting the entire body.

T-Cell: An immune system cell or lymphocyte that directs an immune response to malignant or infected cells.

Testes: Two male reproductive glands located inside the scrotum. The testes are the primary sources for testosterone. Also called testicles.

Testosterone: A male sex hormone chiefly produced by the testicles.

Thrombotic: Causing or relating to blood clotting.

TNM Staging: The most widely used classification system for evaluating the extent of prostate cancer. TNM refers to tumor, nodes and metastases. See Staging.

Transrectal: Through the rectum.

Transurethral: Through the urethra.

Transrectal Ultrasonography: See Ultrasound.

Transurethral Resection of the Prostate (TURP): A surgical procedure to remove tissue obstructing the urethra. The technique involves the insertion of an instrument called a resectoscope into the penile urethra, and is intended to relieve obstruction of urine flow due to enlargement of the prostate.

Tumor: An excessive growth of cells that is caused by uncontrolled and disorderly cell replacement. Abnormal tissue growth may be benign or malignant. See also Benign, Malignant.

TURP: See Transurethral Resection of the Prostate.

Ultrasound (Transrectal Ultrasonography): A painless, non-invasive diagnostic imaging technique using sound waves to create an echo pattern that reveals the structure of organs and tissues. It does not use x-rays.

Understaging: An overly low assessment of clinical stage at diagnosis.

Urethra: The tube that carries urine from the bladder and semen from the prostate out of the body through the penis.

Urologist: A physician who specializes in the diagnosis and the medical and surgical treatment of problems in the urinary and male reproductive systems.

USPIO: This technology uses ultrasmall superparamagnetic iron oxide (USPIO) as an MRI contrast agent for the identification of cancer metastasis in lymph nodes.

Vasectomy: A surgical procedure to render a man sterile by cutting the vas deferens, thus eliminating the passage of sperm from the testes to the prostate.

Vasoactive: Causing the dilation or constriction of blood vessels.

Vesicle: A small sac containing fluid, as in seminal vesicles.

Whitmore-Jewett Staging: A classification system for evaluating the extent of prostate cancer. This system is less widely used for the designation of stage than is TNM staging.

X-rays: High energy radiation that can be used at low levels of intensity to make images of the body's internal structures, or at high intensity for radiation therapy.

THE
WARNING SIGNS
OF PROSTATE CANCER

There are often no warning signs of prostate cancer. In some cases the following symptoms may indicate the presence of the disease. However, please be aware that these symptoms may also be due to benign conditions of the prostate, or other conditions entirely unrelated to prostate cancer:

- ✔ Elevated or rising PSA
- ✔ Abnormal Digital Rectal Exam
- ✔ Blood in urine
- ✔ Pain or difficulty urinating
- ✔ Increased urge to urinate, especially at night
- ✔ Hesitant or intermittent urinary flow
- ✔ Pain or discomfort in area of prostate
- ✔ Unusual and unexplained weight loss
- ✔ Continual pain in lower back, hips or pelvis
- ✔ Increased voiding urgency
- ✔ Inability to urinate
- ✔ Trouble having or keeping an erection (erectile dysfunction)
- ✔ Weakness or numbness in the legs or feet

ABOUT THE
AUTHOR

Michael J. Dattoli, MD

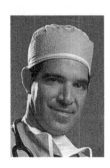

Michael J. Dattoli, MD, is a board-certified radiation oncologist with well over two decades of brachytherapy experience and has performed thousands of prostate implant procedures. He is considered the foremost pioneer in the field, optimizing brachytherapy designs to maximize tumor eradication and minimize symptoms. He has also been the leading trailblazer in the development of Dynamic Adaptive Radiotherapy (DART), utilizing all of the state-of-the-art modalities associated with 4-Dimensional Image-Guided Intensity Modulated Radiotherapy (3D-IMRT). Dr. Dattoli has successfully applied the same technologies to other forms of cancer, including breast, head and neck, GI, GYN, sarcomas and lung malignancies. He is a noted author and speaker in this complex field of medicine.

Dr. Dattoli attended the University of California at Berkeley and was the Valedictorian of his class at Vassar College; he earned his medical degree at Mount Sinai School of Medicine, Radiation Oncology at New York University Medical Center, then distinguished himself at Memorial Sloan-Kettering Cancer Center and New York Hospital-Cornell University Medical Center, as the Special Fellow in Brachytherapy. He was appointed Associate Professor in Brachytherapy and Radiation Oncology at Memorial Sloan- Kettering Cancer Center in New York and at New York Hospital-Cornell University Medical Center prior to relocating to Florida.

Dr. Dattoli also serves on multiple journal editorial review boards. Government appointments include "The Prostate Cancer Task Force" in Florida and consultant to the "Washington Oncology Roundtable Advisory Committee". He was selected by the International Association of Oncologists as a Leading Physician of the World and top Brachytherapist.

THE DATTOLI
CANCER FOUNDATION
MISSION

The Dattoli Cancer Foundation, sponsor of the Prostate Cancer Resource Network, is a 501(c)(3), tax-exempt charitable organization, whose mission is

◆ to raise awareness of the wide-spread incidence of Prostate Cancer and the need for early and annual screenings;

◆ to provide information and support to men newly diagnosed with Prostate Cancer as well as to those with recurrent Prostate Cancer, and

◆ to foster research into better diagnostic tools and treatment options for Prostate Cancer.

Gifts to the Dattoli Foundation make possible publications like this one, and are welcomed anytime. A copy of the official registration and financial information may be obtained from the Division of Consumer Services by calling toll-free (800-435-7352) within the state. Registration does not imply endorsement, approval or recommendations by the state.

Dattoli Cancer Foundation
2803 Fruitville Road
Sarasota, FL 34237
941/365-5599
800/915-1001
fax: 941/330-2317
www.dattolifoundation.org

ORDER
MORE BOOKLETS
IN THE SERIES

This *Prostate Cancer Essentials for Survival* booklet was published by the Datolli Cancer Foundation. For a complete list of booklets in the series and ordering information, please visit the Dattoli Cancer Center Book Shelf at dattoli.com/book-shelf. Current titles include::

✔ *Conquering Prostate Cancer with DART and Brachytherapy*

✔ *The Dattoli Prostate Cancer Challenge: Evaluating All Your Treatment Options*

✔ *The Facts: Comparing Prosate Cancer Treatment Options*

✔ *Interpreting Your PSA Results and Related Prostate Cancer Lab Tests*

✔ *Dynamic Adaptive Radiotherapy*

✔ *Image-Guided Prostate Biopsy: When, Why and What to Expect*

✔ *Dosimetry and Prostate Cancer Radiotherapy*

✔ *Advanced Imaging for Prostate Cancer: A Primer on 3D Color-Flow Power Doppler Ultrasound, Multiparametric MRI and CT Fusion Techniques*

✔ *Radiation Safety and Prostate Cancer: Need You Be Concerned?*

✔ *Hormonal Therapy for Prostate Cancer: The Benefits and Risks*

✔ *Lymph Node Positive Prostate Cancer: Advanced Diagnostics and Treatment*

✔ *The Dattoli Blue Ribbon Prostate Cancer Solution: How to Survive and Thrive Without Surgery*